THE

DETOX

DWELLING

A Practical Guide to Nontoxic Cleaning for Healthier Homes and Greener Living

THE
DETOX
DWELLING

A Practical Guide to Nontoxic Cleaning for
Healthier Homes and Greener Living

By
CATHY MAILS

Published by Smart Publishing
smartpublishingservices.com

Cover Design by Mubbii Designs
Book Formatting by Saqib Arshad
Edited by Renee Lautermilch

The information provided in this book is for educational and informational purposes only. The author and publisher have made every effort to ensure that the content is accurate and up-to-date; however, they make no warranties, express or implied, regarding the completeness, reliability, or effectiveness of the methods, recipes, or recommendations contained herein.

The author and publisher disclaim any liability for any direct, indirect, incidental, or consequential damages resulting from the use or misuse of the information in this book. Readers are encouraged to use their best judgment and consult professionals as needed, especially if they have specific health conditions, allergies, or concerns about using certain ingredients.

Additionally, while many of the cleaning solutions and techniques described in this book are intended to be safe and environmentally friendly, individual results may vary. The author and publisher do not guarantee the performance, safety, or suitability of any product, method, or ingredient for every home or individual. Always conduct a patch test before applying any new cleaning solution to surfaces, and keep all homemade cleaning products out of reach of children and pets.

By using this book, the reader acknowledges and agrees that the responsibility for their own actions, choices, and cleaning practices rests solely with them.

The Detoxed Dwelling: A Practical Guide to Nontoxic Cleaning for Healthier Homes and Greener Living
By Cathy Mails

SMART PUBLISHING

smartpublishingservices.com

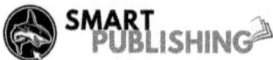

DEDICATION

Growing up, my family and I always recycled, and I learned a lot about caring for the planet. We planted trees and flowers, recycled regularly, and lived near the water in Connecticut. My family was active in the community—participating in the chamber of commerce, Rotary, and other local clubs.

At a very young age, I began my apprenticeship in my parents' business, Madison Cabins, learning the ins and outs of the rental industry. I was frequently exposed to chemical cleaners and developed rashes, even when wearing gloves.

Now that both of my parents have passed, I feel a strong calling to make a difference by educating others about the hidden toxins in their homes.

I dedicate this book to both of my parents, and to my high school friend and fellow author, Christopher Jennings Penders, who encouraged me to write a book after reading my blogs.

TABLE OF CONTENTS

FOREWORD

Some people talk about change. Cathy Mails lives it—in every home she touches, every conversation she has, and now, through the pages you're about to read.

When I first met Cathy at a local networking event, I'll be honest—I was struck by her energy. She was grounded but passionate, tenacious but warm. As we got to know each other better through our shared experiences as small business owners, athletes, and moms, I realized what made her so magnetic: she actually walks the walk. Her mission to create a healthier planet, one home at a time, isn't just something she says—it's how she lives. This book is an incredible extension of her mission, bringing knowledge to so many more homes and touching so many more lives.

The Detox Dwelling is more than a practical guide to non-toxic cleaning. It's Cathy's story—decades of learning, experimenting, and yes, sometimes failing, all in pursuit of healthier living. Her journey from desperately trying to help her child with chemical sensitivities to building North Carolina's only certified green residential cleaning service hasn't been easy. But she's taken all that hard-won knowledge and poured it into these pages. Every room-by-room guide, every step-by-step instruction comes from real experience, tireless hours of research, and buckets of sweat.

Here's what I love about Cathy: she's the real deal. She doesn't just run a green cleaning business—she paddles outrigger canoes to support ocean preservation. She doesn't just talk about sustainability at networking events—she lives it every single day. When she leads her *Sea Green Natural Cleaning* team, you can see her values in action. She's always learning, always growing, always looking for ways to make a bigger impact. Through her daily actions, she educates, empowers, and uplifts others with both compassion and clarity.

I have to say, watching her write this book while juggling everything else— her business, training, competing, family life—has been pretty amazing. Most people would have given up. Yet Cathy never wavered. This book is a true reflection of her passion and purpose, thoughtfully crafted to help others and preserve our precious waters.

As you begin this journey through *The Detox Dwelling*, open these pages ready to transform not just your cleaning routine, but your entire relationship with your home environment. Please read with both curiosity and care. Let this book challenge your habits, awaken your awareness, and empower you to create a home that supports your health and the planet. Whether you're a seasoned green-living advocate or just starting to question what's under your sink, you'll find something here: knowledge, guidance, and compassion. More importantly, you're going to feel empowered to make changes that matter—for your family and for our planet.

This book is truly a gift. And honestly? So is getting to know Cathy Mails. It has been an honor to learn from her and improve the health of my home!

— Brittany Forbes, Physical Therapist, Proud Friend of Cathy Mails, and Fellow Advocate for Healthier Living

INTRODUCTION

To put it bluntly, my mission is to keep this Earth turning as long as possible. Every choice we make has an impact, and for far too long, the way we clean our homes has come at a significant cost to our health and the environment. The manufacture of traditional cleaning products alone requires 6.2 billion pounds of chemicals, many of which are derived from nonrenewable natural resources. The EPA has ranked poor indoor air quality among the top five environmental risks to public health, and their studies show that the toxic chemicals in household cleaners are three times more likely to cause cancer than outdoor air pollution. These statistics are alarming, and for me, they were a wake-up call.

A Life in Cleaning

Cleaning has been a part of my life for as long as I can remember. I grew up managing my parents' business that consisted of six summer rentals and three year-round cottages. The business name was Madison Cabins, located in Madison Connecticut. At the young age of eleven, I began learning all facets of the business—from painting, cleaning, washing laundry, and renting out the units. Later, as an adult, I built a cleaning business, working closely with clients to ensure their homes were both spotless and welcoming. Through these experiences, I became acutely aware of the widespread use of harsh, chemical-laden cleaning products. I saw firsthand how exposure to these products affected people's health—causing skin irritation, respiratory issues, and long-term concerns that many never considered.

For years, I unknowingly used these products myself, assuming that if they were sold on store shelves, they must be safe. But as I learned more about their ingredients and the harm they cause, I knew I could no longer justify using them in my own home, let alone in my clients' homes. That realization was the turning point. I made a commitment to never again expose myself, my family, my pets, or my clients to harmful chemicals. Instead, I founded Sea Green Natural Cleaning, LLC—a company dedicated to using safe, biodegradable, and eco-friendly cleaning products that are manufactured sustainably and do not harm the environment. We only have one planet, and I believe we have a responsibility to protect it.

Why This Book?

I decided to write this book because I know there are many people out there who want a cleaner home without sacrificing their health or the health of the planet. Maybe you're someone who has read about the dangers of conventional cleaning products but doesn't know where to start in making a change. Maybe you're a parent, like me, who wants to create a safer home for your children and pets. Or perhaps you're simply looking for practical, affordable, and effective alternatives to the chemical-laden products that line store shelves. Whatever your reason, this book is for you.

I want to empower you with knowledge and practical solutions. In these pages, I'll share simple, effective, and natural cleaning recipes, tips for creating a healthier home, and insights into why switching to eco-friendly cleaning is one of the best decisions you can make—not just for your household, but for the planet. My goal is to make this transition easy and approachable, proving that you don't need a chemistry degree or a large budget to clean safely and sustainably.

A Small Change Can Make a Big Difference

Margaret Mead once said, "Never doubt that a small group of thoughtful, committed citizens can change the world; indeed, it is the only thing that ever has." I truly believe this to be true. By making small, mindful changes in our own homes, we contribute to a much larger movement toward sustainability. And when enough of us take action, we can drive meaningful change.

So whether you're here out of curiosity or a deep commitment to a healthier lifestyle, I welcome you on this journey. Together, we can redefine what it means to have a truly clean home—one that is safe, natural, and in harmony with the world around us.

How This Book is Structured

This book is divided into three parts, each designed to guide you through a complete transformation in how you clean your home:

Part 1: Understanding Eco-Friendly Cleaning

We'll begin by exploring why making the switch to natural cleaning products is important. You'll learn about the harmful effects of conventional cleaners, the benefits of natural alternatives, and the key ingredients and tools you'll need to get started.

Part 2: Room-by-Room Cleaning Guide

This section provides a step-by-step approach to cleaning every part of your home using safe, effective, and eco-friendly methods. From the bathroom and kitchen to floors, laundry, and even outdoor spaces, you'll find targeted solutions for maintaining a clean and toxin-free living environment.

Part 3: Labels, Ingredients & Sustainability

To help you make informed choices beyond this book, we'll discuss how to read product labels, avoid greenwashing, and recognize toxic ingredients. Additionally, we'll provide DIY cleaning recipes and tips for reducing waste and embracing long-term sustainability in your cleaning routine.

By the end of this book, you'll have the knowledge and tools to maintain a spotless, healthy home without compromising the well-being of your family or the environment. Let's get started!

PART 1

Understanding Eco-Friendly Cleaning

CHAPTER 1

Why Go Green?

The Hidden Dangers of Conventional Cleaners

Every day, we use household cleaners to keep our homes fresh and sanitary, but what if those very products are doing more harm than good? Many conventional cleaning products contain harsh chemicals that can affect indoor air quality, irritate skin, and even contribute to long-term health issues. From respiratory problems to hormone disruption, the chemicals in everyday cleaners can have far-reaching consequences.

Health Risks

> **Respiratory Issues:** Many cleaning sprays release volatile organic compounds (VOCs) that can trigger allergies, asthma, and other respiratory problems.[1]

> **Skin Irritation:** Ingredients like ammonia and bleach can cause skin burns and irritation.[2]

> **Hormone Disruptors:** Some cleaning products contain phthalates and triclosan, which are linked to hormonal imbalances and reproductive health concerns.[3]

Environmental Impact

> **Water Pollution:** Chemicals from cleaning products enter water systems, harming marine life and contaminating drinking water.[4]

> **Air Pollution:** Aerosol sprays and chemical-based deodorizers release toxins into the air, contributing to indoor and outdoor air pollution.[5]

> » **Plastic Waste:** Many cleaning products come in single-use plastic
> bottles, adding to landfill waste and pollution.[6]

The Benefits of Eco-Friendly Cleaning

Going green with your cleaning routine isn't just a trend—it's a healthier, more sustainable way to care for your home and the planet. By switching to natural alternatives, you reduce exposure to harmful chemicals, lower your carbon footprint, and even save money.

Healthier Home Environment

> » Reduces exposure to toxic chemicals.
> » Improves indoor air quality by eliminating synthetic fragrances and VOCs.[7]
> » Safe for children and pets, who are more vulnerable to chemical exposure.

Better for the Planet

> » Biodegradable ingredients break down naturally without polluting waterways.[8]
> » Less reliance on single-use plastics through reusable bottles and DIY solutions.[9]
> » Supports sustainability by reducing chemical runoff into the environment.

Cost-Effective & Simple

> » Many natural ingredients like vinegar, baking soda, and lemon are inexpensive and multipurpose.[10]
> » DIY cleaning recipes allow you to make effective cleaners at a fraction of the cost of store-bought options.

Making the Switch: Small Changes, Big Impact

Transitioning to eco-friendly cleaning doesn't have to be overwhelming. Start by swapping out a few key products and gradually incorporate more sustainable habits into your routine.

Easy First Steps:

1. **Replace One Cleaner at a Time:** Swap chemical-laden all-purpose cleaners for a homemade mix of vinegar and water.
2. **Ditch Synthetic Air Fresheners:** Use essential oils or homemade sprays to freshen up your space without toxins.
3. **Choose Refillable or Reusable Products:** Opt for glass spray bottles and refillable cleaning solutions instead of single-use plastics.

By taking these simple steps, you'll not only create a healthier home but also contribute to a cleaner, greener planet. The journey to eco-friendly cleaning starts here, and the benefits will last for generations to come.

Chapter Notes

1. Zock, J. P., Plana, E., Jarvis, D., Antó, J. M., Kromhout, H., Kennedy, S. M., ... & Kogevinas, M. (2007). The use of household cleaning sprays and adult asthma: an international longitudinal study. American Journal of Respiratory and Critical Care Medicine, 176(8), 735-741.
2. Wolkoff, P., Schneider, T., Kildesø, J., Degerth, R., Jaroszewski, M., & Schunk, H. (1998). Risk in cleaning: chemical and physical exposure. Science of the Total Environment, 215(1-2), 135-156.
3. Dann, A. B., & Hontela, A. (2011). Triclosan: environmental exposure, toxicity and mechanisms of action. Journal of Applied Toxicology, 31(4), 285-311.
4. Warhurst, A. M. (1995). An environmental assessment of alkylphenol ethoxylates and alkylphenols. Journal of Applied Ecology, 32(3), 703-707.
5. Nazaroff, W. W., & Weschler, C. J. (2004). Cleaning products and air fresheners: exposure to primary and secondary air pollutants. Atmospheric Environment, 38(18), 2841-2865

6. Rochman, C. M., Browne, M. A., Halpern, B. S., Hentschel, B. T., Hoh, E., Karapanagioti, H. K., ... & Rios-Mendoza, L. M. (2013). Policy: Classify plastic waste as hazardous. Nature, 494(7436), 169-171.

7. Holmes, D. (2023). 21 Eco-Friendly Cleaning Products You Should Use ASAP. Architectural Digest. Retrieved from https://www.architecturaldigest.com/story/eco-friendly-cleaning-products

8. Green cleaning. (2024). In Wikipedia. Retrieved from https://en.wikipedia.org/wiki/Green_cleaning

9. 7 Simple Ways to Go Green with Your Cleaning Routine. (2022). Better Homes & Gardens. Retrieved from https://www.bhg.com/homekeeping/house-cleaning/tips/eco-friendly-cleaning-ideas/

10. The ultimate guide to non-toxic cleaning products. (2025). Homes & Gardens. Retrieved from https://www.homesandgardens.com/solved/ultimate-shopping-guide-non-toxic-cleaning-supplies

CHAPTER 2

Essential Ingredients for a Healthy Home

Essential Supplies for Green Cleaning

To transition to a healthier home, it's essential to stock up on key natural ingredients that serve multiple cleaning purposes. These household staples are non-toxic, cost-effective, and easy to use.

Must-Have Natural Ingredients

1. **Baking Soda:** A powerful deodorizer, mild abrasive, and stain remover.[1]
2. **White Vinegar:** Excellent for cutting grease, removing odors, and disinfecting surfaces.[2]
3. **Lemon Juice:** Natural antibacterial properties and a fresh, clean scent.[3]
4. **Castile Soap:** A gentle yet effective all-purpose cleaner that is widely available in various stores and online retailers.[4]
5. **Hydrogen Peroxide:** A safe alternative to bleach for disinfecting and stain removal.[5]
6. **Essential Oils (Tea Tree, Lavender, Lemon, Eucalyptus, etc.)** – Adds fragrance and antimicrobial benefits.[6]
7. **Cornstarch:** Useful for polishing furniture and absorbing moisture.
8. **Salt:** Acts as a natural scrubbing agent and disinfectant.[7]
9. **Rubbing Alcohol:** Great for glass cleaning and disinfecting surfaces.

10. **Washing Soda:** A stronger version of baking soda, ideal for heavy-duty cleaning.[8]
11. **Bon Ami:** A gentle yet effective powdered cleanser known for its non-toxic, biodegradable formula.[9]

Why These Ingredients Work

Each of these ingredients serves a specific role in natural cleaning, replacing the need for harsh commercial cleaners that can pose health risks.

> » **Baking soda** neutralizes odors and removes grime without scratching surfaces.
> » **White vinegar** cuts through grease and kills bacteria while being completely safe for pets and children.
> » **Lemon juice** naturally disinfects and removes stains, leaving a pleasant citrus scent.
> » **Castile soap** is a versatile, plant-based soap that works for everything from dishwashing to laundry.
> » **Hydrogen peroxide** disinfects without the toxic fumes of traditional bleach. Note that although it is a powerful and effective natural disinfectant, it can cause damage or discoloration to certain surfaces over time, particularly porous materials like granite, marble, or some types of wood. It may also bleach fabrics and upholstery. Always spot test in an inconspicuous area before applying widely, and store hydrogen peroxide in a dark container to preserve its effectiveness. Use with caution and proper ventilation.
> » **Essential oils** enhance the cleaning power of homemade solutions while providing a natural fragrance.
> » **Bon Ami** is designed to clean a variety of household surfaces without harsh chemicals or scratching delicate materials.

How to Use These Ingredients

> **All-Purpose Cleaner:** Mix equal parts vinegar and water in a spray bottle. Add a few drops of essential oil for fragrance.

> **Glass & Mirror Cleaner:** Combine 1 cup water, 1 cup vinegar, and 1 tablespoon cornstarch for a streak-free shine.

> **Scrubbing Paste:** Make a paste of baking soda and water for cleaning sinks, tubs, and tile grout.

> **Disinfecting Spray:** Mix hydrogen peroxide with water in a spray bottle for a non-toxic disinfectant.

> **Carpet Deodorizer:** Sprinkle baking soda over carpets, let sit for 15 minutes, then vacuum.

> **Bon Ami:** Wet the Surface and lightly dampen the area you want to clean. Apply a small amount of powder directly onto the surface or a damp cloth/sponge. Use a soft cloth, sponge, or non-abrasive brush to scrub the area. Rinse with water and wipe dry to avoid residue.

By keeping these natural ingredients on hand, you'll be equipped to clean every area of your home safely and effectively while reducing your environmental footprint. And if you ever find yourself wondering about the safety of a store-bought product, the Yuka mobile app is a great tool for scanning labels and making informed, healthier choices for your household.

Chapter Notes

1. Arm & Hammer. (n.d.). Baking soda cleaning hacks.
   https://www.armandhammer.com/en/articles/baking-soda-cleaning-hacks
2. Sansoni, B. (2024, March 6). 10 things you can — and can't — clean with vinegar. The Washington Post.
   https://www.washingtonpost.com/home/2024/03/06/cleaning-with-vinegar-dos-donts/

3. WebMD. (n.d.). Lemon: Health benefits and nutrition.
   https://www.webmd.com/diet/health-benefits-lemon

4. Dr. Bronner's. (n.d.). How to make your own all-purpose cleaner.
   https://www.drbronner.com/pages/how-make-natural-all-purpose-cleaner

5. Healthline. (n.d.). Rubbing alcohol vs. hydrogen peroxide for disinfecting.
   https://www.healthline.com/health/rubbing-alcohol-vs-hydrogen-peroxide

6. Healthline. (n.d.). Antibacterial essential oils: How do they work?.
   https://www.healthline.com/health/antibacterial-essential-oils

7. Treehugger. (n.d.). 6 ways to clean your home with salt.
   https://www.treehugger.com/ways-clean-your-home-salt-4856399

8. Arm & Hammer. (n.d.). Super washing soda usage instructions.
   https://www.armandhammer.com/en/articles/super-washing-soda-usage-directions

9. Bon Ami. (n.d.). Bon Ami powder cleanser 14 oz.
   https://www.bonami.com/products/bon-ami-powder-cleanser/

CHAPTER 3

Tools of the Trade

Essential Cleaning Tools for an Eco-Friendly Home

Just as important as the ingredients you use are the tools that help you clean efficiently and sustainably. Investing in the right tools ensures a deeper clean while reducing waste and environmental impact.

Must-Have Cleaning Tools

> **Microfiber Cloths:** Reusable, highly absorbent, and great for dusting and polishing.[1]
> **Glass Spray Bottles:** Durable and reusable for DIY cleaning solutions.[2]
> **Scrub Brushes (with Natural Bristles):** Effective for deep cleaning without scratching surfaces.
> **Sponges (Biodegradable or Reusable):** A sustainable alternative to disposable sponges.[3]
> **Bamboo Cleaning Cloths:** A compostable, eco-friendly substitute for paper towels.
> **Mop with Washable Pads:** Reduces waste compared to disposable mop heads.[4]
> **Vacuum with HEPA Filter:** Helps trap dust and allergens for better air quality.[5]
> **Bucket & Squeegee:** Useful for windows, mirrors, and floor cleaning.
> **Reusable Duster:** A washable duster that captures dust instead of spreading it.
> **Compostable Trash Bags:** An eco-friendly alternative to traditional plastic bags.

Sustainable Cleaning Practices

>> **Choose Durable Over Disposable:** Investing in long-lasting tools cuts down on landfill waste.

>> **Wash & Reuse:** Many cleaning tools can be washed and reused instead of being discarded after a single use.

>> **Opt for Natural Materials:** Tools made from bamboo, recycled plastics, and natural fibers are better for the planet.

By assembling a toolkit with these essential items, you can keep your home clean while making a positive impact on the environment.

The 20/10 Rule: Your Secret Weapon for Saner Cleaning Sessions

Okay, so it's not something you can stash under your sink or add to your spray bottle—but the **20/10 rule** is still one of the most useful "tools" in your eco-friendly cleaning kit.

This simple method involves cleaning for 20 minutes, then taking a 10-minute break to rest, reset, or reward yourself. It's a powerful way to stay productive without getting burned out—especially helpful when you're trying to maintain a clean, healthy home in the middle of a busy life.

How It Works:

>> **20 Minutes On:** Set a timer and choose a specific task—like wiping down the kitchen counters, organizing a drawer, or scrubbing the tub. For those 20 minutes, go all in.

>> **10 Minutes Off:** When the timer rings, stop. Seriously—stop. Step away and do something enjoyable: stretch, sip tea, read a chapter of your book, or just sit down and breathe.

> ❯ **Repeat as Needed:** Stack as many 20/10 cycles as you like. It's great for larger projects, or even for making a dent in everyday messes when time feels tight.

Why It Works:

> ❯ Keeps you from feeling overwhelmed
> ❯ Turns cleaning into manageable chunks
> ❯ Builds in moments of rest (which we all need!)
> ❯ Helps shift your mindset from "perfect" to "progress"

Make It Your Own:

The beauty of the 20/10 rule is how flexible it is. Need shorter bursts? Try 10/5. Want a longer sprint with a bigger break? Go for 30/15. The idea is to pace yourself and keep cleaning from becoming something you dread.

It's not a product or a scrub brush—but this time-based method might just be one of the most valuable tools in your healthy home routine.

Chapter Notes

1. Wikipedia contributors. (2023, December 8). Microfiber. Wikipedia. https://en.wikipedia.org/wiki/Microfiber
2. FastKlean. (n.d.). *6 Must Have Eco-Friendly Cleaning Tools*. https://www.fastklean.co.uk/blog/eco-friendly-cleaning-tips/6-must-have-eco-friendly-cleaning-tools/
3. Epicurious. (2016, March 17). The Cult Cleaning Tools From Iris Hantverk You Need in Your Kitchen. https://www.epicurious.com/expert-advice/iris-hantverk-cleaning-tools-article
4. The Spruce. (2025, May 13). Why You Should Ditch Your Mop and Use This Underrated Cleaning Tool Instead, Pros Say. https://www.thespruce.com/regular-mop-vs-microfiber-mop-11732128
5. Wikipedia contributors. (2025, April 29). Hypoallergenic vacuum cleaner. Wikipedia. https://en.wikipedia.org/wiki/Hypoallergenic_vacuum_cleaner

PART 2

Room-by-Room Cleaning Guide

CHAPTER 4

Bathroom: A Chemical-Free Clean

Introduction

The bathroom is one of the most frequently used spaces in any home, but it is also one of the most chemically treated. Many conventional cleaners contain harsh chemicals that can be harmful to both human health and the environment. Fortunately, there are many natural and eco-friendly alternatives that effectively clean without exposing your household to toxins. This chapter will guide you through creating a healthier bathroom using common, safe ingredients.

Avoiding Harmful Chemicals

Many commercial bathroom cleaners contain toxic ingredients that can be harmful to your health. Here are some to avoid:

> **Hydrochloric Acid:** Common in toilet cleaners; causes respiratory irritation and skin burns.
> - **Respiratory Irritation:** Hydrochloric acid can release toxic fumes that irritate the respiratory system, especially in poorly ventilated areas.
> - **Skin and Eye Damage:** Direct contact with hydrochloric acid can cause severe burns to the skin and eyes. Inhaling the fumes can lead to coughing, choking, and shortness of breath.[1]

- o **Toxic to Pets:** Pets, especially cats and dogs, are at risk of poisoning if they come into contact with hydrochloric acid residues on the floor or drink water contaminated by the chemical.[2]

» **Bleach:** Releases toxic fumes, especially when mixed with other cleaners.

- o **Respiratory Issues:** Inhalation of bleach vapors can cause irritation to the lungs, eyes, and throat, potentially leading to respiratory distress, coughing, and asthma-like symptoms.[3]
- o **Toxicity to Pets:** If pets ingest bleach, it can lead to gastrointestinal distress, including vomiting and diarrhea. It can also cause skin irritation if they come into contact with it.[4]
- o **Chemical Reactions:** When bleach is mixed with other cleaning agents, such as ammonia or acids, it can produce toxic chloramine vapors, which are highly hazardous to human health.[5]

» **Phthalates:** Found in synthetic fragrances; disrupt hormones.

- o **Hormonal Disruption:** Phthalates are endocrine disruptors that can interfere with hormone systems, particularly in developing children. They have been linked to reproductive and developmental issues.[6]
- o **Toxicity to Pets:** Pets who are exposed to phthalates can experience hormone disruption, liver damage, and behavioral changes.[7]

» **Triclosan:** Used in antibacterial soaps; linked to antibiotic resistance.[8, 9]

Toxic Shower Curtains

Many vinyl shower curtains contain harmful chemicals, such as phthalates and organotins, which can off-gas into the air and pose serious health risks, including respiratory issues, hormonal disruption, and neurological damage.[10] These toxins are not chemically bonded to the material, making them more likely to evaporate or cling to household dust, increasing exposure. Research has shown that these chemicals can also contaminate waterways, harming both human health and wildlife.[11]

To reduce exposure to these toxins, consumers should avoid PVC (polyvinyl chloride) shower curtains and instead opt for safer alternatives, such as those made from cotton, polyester, or nylon.[12, 13] Many major retailers have phased out PVC-based curtains, but they can still be found in some stores. When selecting a shower curtain, look for labels that explicitly state "PVC-free" or choose fabric options that can be washed and reused, offering both a healthier and more sustainable choice for your home.

Shower Heads: A Word of Caution

Shower heads can harbor bacteria, mold, and mineral buildup, which may contribute to skin, eye, and ear infections. Over time, warm, moist environments inside showerheads create the perfect breeding ground for harmful microbes like Mycobacterium avium, Pseudomonas aeruginosa, and fungal spores.[14, 15]

How Infections Can Occur:

> **Skin Infections:** Bacteria-laden water droplets can cause irritation, rashes, or folliculitis, especially for those with sensitive skin or weakened immune systems.

> **Eye Infections:** Contaminated water can enter the eyes, potentially causing redness, irritation, or conjunctivitis (pink eye).

> **Ear Infections:** Water containing bacteria may become trapped in the ear canal, increasing the risk of swimmer's ear or other infections.[16]

Prevention Tips:

> **Clean Shower Heads Regularly:** Soak in vinegar or hydrogen peroxide every 1–2 months to kill bacteria.
> **Use a Filtered Showerhead:** Filters reduce mineral buildup and bacteria growth.
> **Run Water Before Use:** Let the water flow for 30 seconds before showering, especially if the shower hasn't been used in a while.

Consistent cleaning and maintenance can significantly reduce the risk of these infections.

Harmful Hand Soap

The Dangers of Antibacterial Soaps: Harmful Ingredients & Health Risks

Many antibacterial hand soaps contain chemicals that pose risks to human health and the environment. While these products are marketed as essential for hygiene, studies suggest they may do more harm than good.

Harmful Ingredients in Antibacterial Soaps & Their Dangers

> **Triclosan & Triclocarban**
  o **Endocrine Disruptors:** Mimic hormones, potentially affecting reproductive health, sperm quality, and thyroid function.
  o **Immune System Effects:** Linked to increased allergies and hay fever, particularly in children.[17]
  o **Environmental Impact:** These chemicals do not break down easily, polluting water systems and harming aquatic life.[18]

> **Phthalates**
>> o **Hormone Disruptors:** Can interfere with reproductive development and increase the risk of certain cancers.[19]
>> o **Absorption Risk:** Found in synthetic fragrances, phthalates can enter the body through the skin.[20]

> **Sodium Lauryl Sulfate (SLS)**
>> o **Skin Irritation:** Causes dryness, irritation, and worsens conditions like eczema.[21]
>> o **Toxin Exposure:** Often contaminated with 1,4-dioxane, a potential carcinogen.[22]

> **Antibacterial Resistance**
>> o Overuse of antibacterial products can contribute to bacterial resistance, making some strains harder to eliminate with antibiotics.[23]
>> o Studies show that antibacterial soap is not more effective than regular soap at reducing bacteria.[24]

Healthier Alternatives to Conventional Antibacterial Soaps

Switching to natural soaps eliminates exposure to harmful chemicals while still maintaining cleanliness and hygiene.

> **Castile Soap**
>> o **What It Is:** A gentle, plant-based soap made from natural oils like olive, coconut, or hemp.
>> o **Why It's Safer:** Free of synthetic fragrances, biodegradable, and non-toxic.[25]
>> o **How to Use:** Dilute with water for liquid hand soap or use in a foaming dispenser.

> **Liquid Coconut Oil Soap**
>   o **What It Is:** Made from saponified coconut oil, providing natural cleansing and moisture.
>   o **Why It's Safer:** Gentle on skin, antimicrobial, and free from synthetic chemicals.[26]

> **Aloe Vera Hand Soap**
>   o **What It Is:** A soothing soap infused with aloe vera for sensitive skin.
>   o **Why It's Safer:** Aloe is naturally moisturizing and has antibacterial properties.[27]

> **Essential Oils for Natural Cleansing**
>   o **Tea Tree Oil:** Antimicrobial and antifungal.[28]
>   o **Lavender Oil:** Soothes skin and has antibacterial properties.[29]
>   o **Lemon Oil:** Cuts grease and has antiviral benefits.[30]
>   o **Peppermint Oil:** Refreshing and antimicrobial.[31]

DIY All-Natural Hand Soap Recipe

This homemade liquid soap is free from harsh chemicals and can be customized with essential oils.

Ingredients:

> 1 cup liquid Castile soap
> 1 tablespoon carrier oil (almond, jojoba, or coconut oil)
> 10-15 drops of essential oil (tea tree, lavender, eucalyptus, etc.)

Instructions:

> Mix all ingredients in a soap dispenser.
> Shake well before use.
> Use as a regular hand soap, enjoying a toxin-free alternative!

Making informed choices about the products you use in your home can significantly reduce exposure to harmful chemicals and protect both your health and the environment. By avoiding toxic ingredients in bathroom cleaners, shower curtains, and hand soaps, you can create a safer, more sustainable living space. Opting for natural alternatives, such as Castile soap and essential oils, not only minimizes health risks but also supports eco-friendly practices. Small changes in your cleaning and hygiene routine can have a lasting impact, ensuring a healthier home for you, your family, and even your pets.

Natural Cleaning Ingredients & Their Uses

So, what's the alternative to using harmful chemicals? There are fortunately a lot of natural cleaning ingredients that are both safe and effective. Here are a few along with their uses.

Baking Soda

> » **Deodorizer:** Absorbs odors in trash cans, drains, and even bathroom rugs.
> » **Scrubbing Paste:** Mix with water to create a paste for scrubbing sinks, tubs, and countertops.
> » **Stain Remover:** Effective against soap scum and hard water stains.
> » **Toilet Cleaner:** Sprinkle into the toilet bowl and scrub to remove stains.

White Vinegar

> » **Disinfectant:** Works well for sanitizing sinks, counters, and tubs.
> » **Limescale Remover:** Breaks down mineral deposits on faucets, showerheads, and glass doors.
> » **Toilet Cleaner:** Pour into the toilet and let sit for 10-15 minutes before scrubbing.

> **Soap Scum Fighter:** Mix with baking soda for an effective tub and tile cleaner.

Lemon Juice

> **Stain Remover:** Ideal for removing rust stains from sinks and tubs.
> **Deodorizer:** Neutralizes odors and leaves a fresh scent.
> **Metal Polish:** Mix with baking soda to shine and clean faucets and fixtures.

Castile Soap

> **All-Purpose Cleaner:** Dilute with water to clean sinks, counters, and tubs.
> **Shower Cleaner:** Mix with vinegar or lemon juice for tile and grout cleaning.
> **Dish Soap Substitute:** Gentle enough to use for washing small bathroom accessories.

Bon Ami

> **Bathtubs and Showers:** Removes soap scum, mildew stains, and hard water deposits.
> **Toilets:** Cleans ceramic surfaces and leaves a fresh shine.
> **Tile and Grout:** Gently scrubs grout lines without damaging tiles.

Hydrogen Peroxide

> **Disinfectant:** Sanitizes toilet handles, sinks, and faucets.
> **Mold & Mildew Remover:** Spray on moldy surfaces, let sit, then scrub.
> **Stain Remover:** Lifts stains from towels and shower curtains.

Essential Oils (Tea Tree, Lavender, Lemon, Eucalyptus, etc.)

> **Disinfectant:** Tea tree oil has natural antibacterial and antifungal properties.
> **Air Freshener:** Add to a diffuser or a spray bottle with water to eliminate odors.
> **Mold Prevention:** Mix with water and wipe down surfaces to deter mold growth.

Salt (Epsom or Table Salt)

> **Drain Cleaner:** Mix with hot water to clear minor blockages.
> **Scrubbing Agent:** Combine with vinegar or baking soda for tough scrubbing jobs.
> **Grout Cleaner:** Use as an abrasive for scrubbing grout lines.

Rubbing Alcohol

> **Mirror & Glass Cleaner:** Mix with water for streak-free shine.
> **Disinfecting Wipes:** Use on bathroom handles and high-touch areas.
> **Mold Spot Treatment:** Apply to mildew-prone spots for extra protection.

Other Household Items with Cleaning Uses

> **Shaving Cream:** Streak-free mirror cleaning and upholstery stain removal.
> **Toothpaste:** Polishing metal fixtures and cleaning grout.
> **Cornstarch, Cornmeal, and Boric Acid:** Other natural agents with unique uses.

Switching to natural cleaning ingredients is an easy and effective way to maintain a clean home without exposing yourself to harmful chemicals.

With common household staples like baking soda, vinegar, and essential oils, you can tackle everything from disinfecting surfaces to removing stains. These natural alternatives are not only safer for your health but also better for the environment. By incorporating them into your cleaning routine, you can create a fresher, healthier space while reducing your reliance on toxic commercial products.

Bathroom Items as Cleaning Tools

In a bind with no cleaning tools on hand and need something fast? Don't worry! Some of the things you can find just sitting around your bathroom actually work great for cleaning the different areas of your bathroom—and they're cheap too!

Old Toothbrush

> » **Uses:**
>> o **Grout Cleaning:** Ideal for scrubbing grout lines or tight corners in your bathroom.
>> o **Faucet & Drain Cleaning:** The small bristles are perfect for cleaning faucet handles, drain covers, and other hard-to-reach areas.
>> o **Detail Cleaning:** Use to clean the corners and edges of sinks, tubs, and toilets.

Old Newspaper

> » **Uses:**
>> o **Window Cleaning:** Use newspaper to clean glass without leaving streaks.
>> o **Mirror Polishing:** Works similarly to microfiber for polishing mirrors and glass.
>> o **Deodorizing:** Crumpled newspaper can be placed in shoes or trash cans to absorb odors.

Toilet Paper Rolls

Empty toilet paper rolls can be repurposed for several creative cleaning tasks.

> **Uses:**
> - o **Dusting:** Use the cardboard roll to clean baseboards or narrow spaces between furniture. Wrap a cloth around it for a DIY dusting tool.
> - o **Organize Cables:** Use toilet paper rolls to organize loose cables or cords that may be cluttering your bathroom or other areas of the house.
> - o **Clean Tight Spaces:** Wrap a cloth around the roll and use it to clean in-between spaces, like air vents or tight corners.

Cotton Balls or Pads

Cotton balls or pads are inexpensive cleaning tools for delicate or detailed cleaning tasks.

> **Uses:**
> - o **Disinfect Small Areas:** Dip a cotton ball in rubbing alcohol or vinegar to clean small spots, such as faucet handles or light switches.
> - o **Clean Small Crevices:** Use them to clean hard-to-reach places like around faucets or the edges of your sink.

Squeegee

A bathroom squeegee is a must-have tool to prevent soap scum and water stains from building up on glass surfaces.

> » **Uses:**
>> o **Clean Shower Doors and Windows:** After every shower, use a squeegee to remove excess water from shower doors or bathroom windows to prevent water spots and mold growth.
>> o **Mirror Cleaning:** Use a squeegee to quickly wipe down mirrors after showers.

Using Q-Tips (Cotton Swabs)

Q-tips have a soft, absorbent cotton tip that can be used for precise cleaning, especially in tight or hard-to-reach areas.

> » **Uses:**
>> o **Cleaning Delicate or Detailed Spots:** Think areas around your faucet and sink

Dental Floss

Dental floss is thin, strong, and flexible, making it ideal for cleaning tight spaces, removing grime, and tackling areas that are difficult to reach with other cleaning tools.

> » **Uses:**
>> o **Super Tight Spaces:** Can't fit a q-tip in there? Try dental floss! It's not just great for cleaning those tight spaces between your teeth—it can be used to clean those tight spaces around your house too!

Repurposing everyday bathroom items as cleaning tools is a smart, budget-friendly way to tackle messes without extra expense. From using an old toothbrush for grout cleaning to repurposing newspaper for streak-free glass, these simple hacks make cleaning easier and more efficient. With a little creativity, you can turn common household items into powerful cleaning tools, saving time and money while keeping your bathroom spotless.

It's Time to Clean! Cleaning Specific Bathroom Areas

Toilet Cleaning

1. Sprinkle baking soda into the bowl.
2. Add 1-2 cups of vinegar and let sit for 10 minutes.
3. Scrub with a toilet brush and flush.
4. For deep cleaning, add a few drops of tea tree oil for extra disinfecting power.

Sink and Countertops

1. Mix equal parts vinegar and water in a spray bottle.
2. Spray on surfaces and wipe clean with a microfiber cloth.
3. For stubborn stains, use a baking soda paste and scrub with an old toothbrush.

Bathtubs and Showers

1. Spray vinegar on soap scum and let sit for 10 minutes.
2. Scrub with baking soda and water paste.
3. Rinse with warm water and wipe down with a squeegee.

Glass and Mirrors

1. Mix one part vinegar with one part rubbing alcohol in a spray bottle.
2. Spray on mirrors and wipe with a microfiber cloth or newspaper for a streak-free shine.

Floors

1. Mix ½ cup vinegar with 1 gallon of warm water.
2. Mop floors with the solution to disinfect and remove grime.
3. For extra shine, add a few drops of lemon essential oil.

Drains

1. Pour ½ cup baking soda down the drain.
2. Gently pour ½ cup vinegar and cover the drain for 30 minutes.
3. Rinse with boiling water to clear clogs and deodorize.

Faucet and Showerhead Care

1. Soak a cloth in vinegar and wrap it around faucets or showerheads to remove mineral deposits.
2. Leave for 1-2 hours, then scrub with an old toothbrush.
3. Rinse with warm water and dry with a microfiber cloth.

Aerator Filter Care

1. Remove the aerator from the faucet and soak it in vinegar for 30–60 minutes to dissolve mineral buildup.
2. Scrub the parts with a baking soda paste and an old toothbrush for stubborn debris.
3. Rinse thoroughly with warm water and reattach the aerator to the faucet.

Sustainable Bathroom Habits

1. Replace disposable cleaning tools with reusable options (microfiber cloths, old toothbrushes).
2. Avoid flushing wipes, even "flushable" ones, as they contribute to clogs and environmental pollution.
3. Use DIY air fresheners instead of synthetic sprays.

Septic System Considerations

1. Avoid "flushable" wipes! People flushing wet wipes down the toilet is the single biggest cause of sewer blockages – in fact, they accounted for 93% of the matter. Most Wipes are not compostable or biodegradable.[32]

2. Your septic system contains a living collection of organisms that digest and treat waste.

3. Avoid using or flushing household chemicals that can disrupt the bacteria in your septic system, leading to failure. Harmful chemicals include bleach, antibacterial soaps, and cleaners with synthetic chemicals.

4. As a safer alternative, use vinegar, baking soda, and essential oils.

A chemical-free bathroom is healthier, safer, and just as effective at staying clean and fresh. By using natural ingredients like vinegar, baking soda, and essential oils, you can eliminate grime and bacteria without exposing your household to toxic chemicals. Plus, these solutions are cost-effective and environmentally friendly. Make the switch today for a cleaner, greener home!

Did You Know? Surprising Bathroom Solutions

Hydrogen Peroxide: The "No Questions, Just Clean" Cleaner

Hydrogen peroxide is the multi-tasking hero we all need. It's like that friend who shows up to the party with snacks, drinks, and an extra charger.

Use it on:

> **Whitening grout.** Mix hydrogen peroxide with baking soda and scrub away. Your grout will look like it was installed yesterday!

>> **Cleaning mirrors and glass.** Hydrogen peroxide is a streak-free, shine-giving miracle for mirrors and windows. Just spray it on and wipe with a microfiber cloth. You'll be able to see into the future.

Fun Fact: Hydrogen peroxide is amazing for disinfecting.

Rubbing Alcohol: The Fast and Furious Cleaner

Rubbing alcohol is like a ninja—silent, effective, and fast. If you need something cleaned *yesterday*, rubbing alcohol's your go-to.

Use it on:

>> **Sticky residue removal.** Whether it's tape, glue, or that weird gunk from stickers, rubbing alcohol takes it all off like magic. Just apply some to a cloth and wipe away.

>> **Disinfecting surfaces.** Rubbing alcohol kills germs in record time. Wipe down your kitchen counters, doorknobs, and light switches—just be careful not to use it on certain surfaces like acrylic or painted finishes.

Fun Fact: Rubbing alcohol is like the clean-up crew after a wild party. It's fast, efficient, and doesn't judge you for how much you've spilled.

Chapter Notes

1. Centers for Disease Control and Prevention. (n.d.). Hydrochloric acid. National Institute for Occupational Safety and Health (NIOSH). Retrieved from https://www.cdc.gov/niosh/npg/npgd0339.html
2. Cornelison, K. (2025, January 9). These are the cleaners to avoid around pets. Better Homes & Gardens. Retrieved from https://www.bhg.com/cleaning-ingredients-to-avoid-with-pets-8750716

3. Tru Earth. (n.d.). The dangers of lasting bleach fumes when cleaning the home. Retrieved from https://tru.earth/blogs/tru-living/the-dangers-of-lasting-bleach-fumes-when-cleaning-the-home

4. Cornelison, K. (2025, January 9). These are the cleaners to avoid around pets. Better Homes & Gardens. Retrieved from https://www.bhg.com/cleaning-ingredients-to-avoid-with-pets-8750716

5. Centers for Disease Control and Prevention. (n.d.). Facts about chloramine. Retrieved from https://emergency.cdc.gov/agent/chloramine/basics/facts.asp

6. Wikipedia contributors. (2025, May 10). Endocrine disruptor. Wikipedia. Retrieved from https://en.wikipedia.org/wiki/Endocrine_disruptor

7. Cornelison, K. (2025, January 9). These are the cleaners to avoid around pets. Better Homes & Gardens. Retrieved from https://www.bhg.com/cleaning-ingredients-to-avoid-with-pets-8750716

8. Wikipedia contributors. (2025, April 30). Triclosan. Wikipedia. Retrieved from https://en.wikipedia.org/wiki/Triclosan

9. Park, A. (2014, November 17). This soap ingredient linked to liver tumors in mice. Time. Retrieved from https://time.com/3589572/triclosan-liver-tumors-mice/

10. Los Angeles Times. (2008, June 13). That 'new shower curtain smell'? It's toxic, study says. https://www.latimes.com/archives/la-xpm-2008-jun-13-me-showercurtain13-story.html

11. Center for Health, Environment & Justice. (2008). Volatile Vinyl: The New Shower Curtain's Chemical Smell. https://chej.org/wp-content/uploads/Volatile%20Vinyl%20-%20REP%20008.pdf

12. Ron & Lisa. (2014, February 12). 5 Non-Toxic & PVC-Free Shower Curtain Alternatives. https://ronandlisa.com/5-nontoxic-pvcfree-shower-curtain-alternatives/

13. Dahl, L. (2015, March 2). Non-Toxic Shower Curtains. https://lindsaydahl.com/non-toxic-shower-curtains/

14. Falkinham, J. O., Iseman, M. D., de Haas, P., & van Soolingen, D. (2008). Mycobacterium avium in a shower linked to pulmonary disease. Journal of Water and Health, 6(2), 209–213.

15. Wikipedia contributors. (2025, May 6). Pseudomonas aeruginosa. Wikipedia. https://en.wikipedia.org/wiki/Pseudomonas_aeruginosa

16. University of Washington Department of Environmental & Occupational Health Sciences. (2019, October 22). The bacteria in your shower. https://deohs.washington.edu/hsm-blog/bacteria-your-shower

17. Weatherly, L. M., & Gosse, J. A. (2017). Triclosan exposure, transformation, and human health effects. Journal of Toxicology and Environmental Health, Part B, 20(8), 447–469. https://doi.org/10.1080/10937404.2017.1399306

18. U.S. Food and Drug Administration. (2019, March 19). Antibacterial soap? You can skip it—Use plain soap and water. https://www.fda.gov/consumers/consumer-updates/antibacterial-soap-you-can-skip-it-use-plain-soap-and-water

19. Zota, A. R., Calafat, A. M., & Woodruff, T. J. (2014). Temporal trends in phthalate exposures: Findings from the National Health and Nutrition Examination Survey, 2001–2010. Environmental Health Perspectives, 122(3), 235–241. https://doi.org/10.1289/ehp.1306681

20. Agency for Toxic Substances and Disease Registry. (2022). Toxicological profile for di(2-ethylhexyl)phthalate (DEHP). https://www.atsdr.cdc.gov/toxprofiles/tp9.pdf

21. MedlinePlus. (2022). Sodium lauryl sulfate. U.S. National Library of Medicine. https://medlineplus.gov/ency/article/002749.htm

22. U.S. Department of Health and Human Services. (2020). 1,4-Dioxane. National Toxicology Program. https://ntp.niehs.nih.gov/whatwestudy/topics/dioxane/index.html

23. Aiello, A. E., Larson, E. L., & Levy, S. B. (2007). Consumer antibacterial soaps: Effective or just risky? Clinical Infectious Diseases, 45(Supplement_2), S137–S147. https://doi.org/10.1086/519178

24. Centers for Disease Control and Prevention. (2016, September 2). Q&A: Antibacterial soaps. https://www.cdc.gov/media/releases/2016/p0902-antibacterial-soap.html

25. Dr. Bronner's. (n.d.). Castile soap: A true soap, not a detergent. https://www.drbronner.com/pages/our-products

26. DebMandal, M., & Mandal, S. (2011). Coconut (Cocos nucifera L.: Arecaceae): In health promotion and disease prevention. Asian Pacific Journal of Tropical Medicine, 4(3), 241–247. https://doi.org/10.1016/S1995-7645(11)60078-3

27. Boudreau, M. D., & Beland, F. A. (2006). An evaluation of the biological and toxicological properties of Aloe barbadensis (Miller), Aloe vera. Journal of

Environmental Science and Health, Part C, 24(1), 103–154.
https://doi.org/10.1080/10590500600614303

28. Carson, C. F., Hammer, K. A., & Riley, T. V. (2006). Melaleuca alternifolia (Tea Tree) oil: A review of antimicrobial and other medicinal properties. Clinical Microbiology Reviews, 19(1), 50–62.
https://doi.org/10.1128/CMR.19.1.50-62.2006

29. Cavanagh, H. M. A., & Wilkinson, J. M. (2002). Biological activities of lavender essential oil. Phytotherapy Research, 16(4), 301–308.
https://doi.org/10.1002/ptr.1103

30. Ali, B., Al-Wabel, N. A., Shams, S., Ahamad, A., Khan, S. A., & Anwar, F. (2015). Essential oils used in aromatherapy: A systemic review. Asian Pacific Journal of Tropical Biomedicine, 5(8), 601–611.
https://doi.org/10.1016/j.apjtb.2015.05.007

31. McKay, D. L., & Blumberg, J. B. (2006). A review of the bioactivity and potential health benefits of peppermint tea (Mentha piperita L.). Phytotherapy Research, 20(8), 619–633. https://doi.org/10.1002/ptr.1936

32. Water UK. (2017). Wipes in sewer blockages: A report on the contribution of flushable and non-flushable wipes to sewer blockages.
https://www.water.org.uk/wp-content/uploads/2018/11/Wipes-in-sewer-blockages-2017.pdf

CHAPTER 5

Kitchen: The Heart of Your Home

Avoiding Harmful Chemicals in the Kitchen

The kitchen is the heart of the home, where meals are prepared, families gather, and memories are made. However, many conventional kitchen cleaning products contain harmful chemicals that can pose risks to both health and the environment. By identifying and avoiding these chemicals, you can create a healthier space for cooking and dining.

Common Harmful Chemicals Found in the Kitchen

Many kitchen cleaning tools, such as synthetic sponges, contain harmful chemicals that pose risks to both human health and the environment. Many synthetic sponges, including well-known brands, contain microplastics and potentially toxic substances that can shed plastic particles into waterways and leach harmful chemicals over time.[1] These chemicals include formaldehyde-melamine-sodium bisulfite copolymer, commonly found in melamine foam sponges (often marketed as "magic erasers"), which can irritate the skin and respiratory system.[2] Additionally, synthetic sponges may contain flame retardants, dyes, and other toxic substances that can linger on kitchen surfaces and transfer to food.[3] Choosing biodegradable alternatives, such as natural fiber sponges or plant-based scrubbers, can help reduce exposure to these harmful compounds.[4]

Many commercial cleaning products contain synthetic chemicals that can contribute to indoor air pollution, trigger allergies, and even pose long-term health risks. Here are some of the most common harmful chemicals found in kitchen products:

1. Phthalates

> **Found in:** Air fresheners, dish soaps, and plastic containers
> **Health risks:** Phthalates are endocrine disruptors, meaning they can interfere with hormone function. Prolonged exposure has been linked to reproductive issues and developmental problems in children.[5]

2. Triclosan

> **Found in:** Antibacterial dishwashing liquids and hand soaps
> **Health risks:** Triclosan can contribute to antibiotic resistance and has been linked to thyroid hormone disruption.[6]

3. Ammonia

> **Found in:** Glass cleaners, oven cleaners, and polishing agents
> **Health risks:** Ammonia is a respiratory irritant that can trigger asthma and lung issues. It is particularly dangerous when mixed with bleach, producing toxic fumes.[7]

4. Chlorine

> **Found in:** Bleach, disinfecting sprays, and some dishwashing detergents
> **Health risks:** Chlorine exposure can irritate the skin, eyes, and respiratory system. Long-term exposure has been linked to thyroid disruption.[8]

5. Formaldehyde

> **Found in:** Some dishwashing liquids, household disinfectants, and synthetic sponges

> **Health risks:** Formaldehyde is a known carcinogen and can cause irritation to the respiratory system and skin. It is also present in melamine foam sponges, which release small amounts of formaldehyde when used.[9]

6. Perchloroethylene (PERC)

> **Found in:** Some degreasers and stain removers
> **Health risks:** PERC has been classified as a potential carcinogen and may cause dizziness, nausea, and respiratory issues with prolonged exposure.[10]

7. Sodium Hydroxide

> **Found in:** Oven cleaners and drain cleaners
> **Health risks:** This highly corrosive chemical can cause severe burns to the skin and eyes and is harmful if inhaled.[11]

Eliminating harmful chemicals from your kitchen doesn't mean sacrificing cleanliness. By choosing safer alternatives and being mindful of the products you use, you can maintain a spotless, healthy kitchen while reducing exposure to toxins. Small changes, like switching to non-toxic cleaners and using natural disinfectants, can significantly improve the safety of your home and the well-being of your family.

Healthier Cleaning Alternatives and Found Objects You Can Use for Cleaning in the Kitchen

A clean kitchen doesn't have to come at the cost of your health or the environment. Many conventional cleaning products contain harmful chemicals, but there are natural, safer alternatives that can be just as effective. Additionally, many everyday kitchen items can serve as excellent cleaning tools, reducing waste and reliance on synthetic cleaners.

Natural Cleaning Alternatives

1. Baking Soda

Why it works: Baking soda is a gentle abrasive that helps break down grease and grime while neutralizing odors.

Uses:

- Scrubbing surfaces like countertops, sinks, and stovetops.
- Deodorizing the refrigerator, garbage disposal, and trash cans.
- Removing stains from pots and pans by creating a paste with water.

2. White Vinegar

Why it works: Vinegar is a natural disinfectant that cuts through grease and eliminates bacteria.

Uses:

- Mixing with water for an all-purpose cleaner for countertops and appliances.
- Breaking down mineral deposits in coffee makers and kettles.
- Cleaning glass surfaces for a streak-free shine.
- Cleaning an instant pot.

3. Lemon Juice

Why it works: The acidity of lemons makes them effective at cutting grease and acting as a natural antibacterial agent.

Uses:

- Removing stains from cutting boards and countertops.
- Deodorizing sinks and garbage disposals.
- Polishing brass and copper cookware.

4. Castile Soap

Why it works: A plant-based soap that is non-toxic yet powerful for breaking down dirt and grease.

Uses:

> ❯ Dilute with water for dish soap or surface cleaner.
> ❯ Mixing with baking soda for a powerful scouring paste.

5. Bon Ami

Why it works: a gentle yet effective powdered cleanser known for its non-toxic, biodegradable formula.

Uses:

> ❯ Effectively removes grease, grime, and burnt-on food from stovetops.
> ❯ Great for scrubbing stainless steel, porcelain, and composite sinks without scratching.
> ❯ Safe for most solid surfaces, including granite and quartz.
> ❯ Can help remove stubborn stains and baked-on food from pots and pans.
> ❯ Gently scrubs away grease buildup on glass oven doors.

6. Hydrogen Peroxide

Why it works: A natural disinfectant that is safer than bleach.

Uses:

> ❯ Disinfecting cutting boards and kitchen sponges.
> ❯ Removing stains from countertops and grout.
> ❯ Sanitizing produce when diluted with water.

7. Olive Oil

Why it works: Acts as a natural polish and moisturizer for surfaces.

Uses:

> » Polishing wooden cutting boards and stainless steel appliances.
> » Conditioning cast iron cookware.
> » Removing sticky residue from labels and jars.

8. Essential Oils (Tea Tree, Lavender, Lemon, or Eucalyptus)

Why they work: Essential oils have natural antibacterial and antifungal properties while adding a pleasant scent.

Uses:

> » Adding to homemade cleaning solutions for extra disinfecting power.
> » Mixing with baking soda to create a natural carpet deodorizer.

Found Objects You Can Use for Cleaning

1. Old Toothbrushes

> » Great for scrubbing grout, cleaning around sink fixtures, and removing buildup in hard-to-reach places.

2. Coffee Grounds

> » Used as a gentle abrasive for scrubbing greasy pots and pans.
> » Absorbs odors in the fridge or trash can.

3. Rice

> » Effective for cleaning narrow-necked bottles and vases when shaken with soapy water.

4. Salt

> Works as a natural scouring agent for scrubbing cast iron pans.

> Combined with lemon juice to disinfect cutting boards.

5. Cornstarch

> Can be used as a natural carpet cleaner by absorbing grease stains.

> Works as a glass cleaner when mixed with vinegar and water.

6. Coconut Oil

> Removes sticky residues from surfaces.

> Conditions wooden utensils and cutting boards.

7. Newspaper

> Provides a streak-free way to clean glass and mirrors.

8. Banana Peels

> Can be used to polish silverware and leather surfaces.

9. Aluminum Foil

> Wadded up, it can scrub off burnt food from grills and pans.

Switching to natural cleaning alternatives and repurposing common household items can significantly reduce exposure to harmful chemicals while promoting a more sustainable lifestyle. These simple changes can help keep your kitchen clean and safe while minimizing environmental impact.

It's Time to Clean! Cleaning Specific Kitchen Areas

A clean kitchen is essential for a healthy and inviting home. Each area of the kitchen requires specific cleaning techniques to maintain hygiene and prevent the buildup of bacteria, grease, and odors. Below is a comprehensive guide to cleaning all common kitchen areas efficiently and safely.

1. Oven and Stove

Oven
Cleaning Method:

> » **Baking Soda Paste:** Sprinkle baking soda onto the surface and spray with vinegar to create a paste, spread it over the oven interior, and let it sit overnight. Wipe off with a damp cloth and rinse with white vinegar.
> » **Steam Cleaning:** Place a heat-safe bowl with water and lemon juice inside the oven at 250°F for 30 minutes to loosen grime.
> » **Racks:** Soak in a sink filled with warm water and dish soap, scrub, and rinse.

Stove
Cleaning Method:

> » **Gas Burners:** Remove grates and soak in soapy water. Scrub with baking soda paste and rinse.
> » **Electric Coils:** Wipe with a damp cloth and baking soda; avoid soaking.
> » **Glass Cooktops:** Sprinkle baking soda, spray with vinegar, let sit for 10 minutes, and wipe clean with a microfiber cloth.

2. Sink

Cleaning Method:

> » **Daily Cleaning:** Rinse with hot water and dish soap.
> » **Deep Cleaning:** Sprinkle baking soda over the sink, scrub with a sponge, and rinse with vinegar for a deep clean.
> » **Unclogging Drain:** Pour ½ cup baking soda followed by ½ cup vinegar. Let sit for 15 minutes, then flush with boiling water.

> **Stainless Steel Shine:** Polish with a few drops of olive oil on a soft cloth.

Aerator Filter Care

1. Remove the aerator from the faucet and soak it in vinegar for 30–60 minutes to dissolve mineral buildup.
2. Scrub the parts with a baking soda paste and an old toothbrush for stubborn debris.
3. Rinse thoroughly with warm water and reattach the aerator to the faucet.

3. Garbage Disposal

Cleaning Method:

> **Deodorizing:** Drop ice cubes made of vinegar and lemon juice into the disposal and run it with cold water.
> **Grease Removal:** Pour a small amount of dish soap into the disposal, run cold water, and turn it on.
> **Deep Clean:** Scrub the rubber splash guard with an old toothbrush and soapy water.

4. Dishwasher

Cleaning Method:

> **Daily Maintenance:** Rinse dishes before loading to prevent buildup.
> **Monthly Deep Clean:** Run an empty cycle with a cup of white vinegar on the top rack, then sprinkle baking soda on the bottom and run another short cycle.
> **Filter Cleaning:** Remove and scrub the filter with warm soapy water.

5. Countertops

Cleaning Method:

>> **Daily Cleaning:** Wipe down with warm soapy water or a vinegar-water mix.

>> **Stain Removal:** For stubborn stains, sprinkle baking soda on a damp sponge and gently scrub.

>> **Stone Countertops:** Use a mild soap and water solution; avoid acidic cleaners like vinegar or lemon juice.

6. Cabinets

Cleaning Method:

>> **Grease Removal:** Mix equal parts vinegar and water, wipe cabinets, and dry with a cloth.

>> **Wood Cabinets:** Use a mild dish soap solution and polish with olive oil to maintain shine.

>> **Handles and Knobs:** Wipe with a disinfectant or soapy water weekly.

7. Microwave

Cleaning Method:

>> **Steam Cleaning:** Fill a microwave-safe bowl with water and lemon juice, heat for 5 minutes, and wipe clean.

>> **Exterior Cleaning:** Wipe with a damp cloth and mild dish soap.

>> **Turntable Cleaning:** Remove and wash with warm soapy water.

8. Floors

Cleaning Method:

>> **Daily Sweeping:** Remove crumbs and dust.

> - **Deep Cleaning:** Mop with a mixture of warm water and a few drops of dish soap.
> - **Tile Grout Cleaning:** Scrub with baking soda and a toothbrush for deep stains.

9. Small Appliances (Toaster, Coffee Maker, Blender, etc.)

Cleaning Method:

- **Toaster:** Remove crumbs, wipe exterior with vinegar solution.
- **Coffee Maker:** Run a cycle with vinegar, followed by a water-only cycle to rinse.
- **Blender:** Blend warm soapy water for easy cleaning, then rinse.

No, we didn't forget the fridge!

How to Clean the Inside of a Refrigerator—Naturally

Keeping your refrigerator clean doesn't have to mean using harsh chemicals. With a few simple ingredients like baking soda, white vinegar, and warm water, you can keep your fridge fresh, clean, and food-safe—all without worrying about lingering chemical residues.

What You'll Need:

> - Baking soda
> - White vinegar
> - Warm water
> - Natural dish soap (optional)
> - Clean sponge or cloth
> - Microfiber cloth or towel
> - Small bowl or bucket
> - Toothbrush or small scrub brush (optional)

Step-by-Step Instructions:

1. Empty the Fridge: Take everything out. This gives you full access to all surfaces and prevents any food from being contaminated during cleaning.

2. Remove Shelves and Drawers: Take out any removable parts and wash them separately with warm water and a few drops of natural dish soap. Scrub gently, rinse well, and let them dry.

3. Mix Your Cleaner: In a bowl or bucket, mix one of the following:

> 1 cup warm water + 1 tablespoon baking soda (great for lifting grime and odors)

> 1 cup water + 1 cup white vinegar (naturally antibacterial)

4. Wipe Down the Interior: Dip your sponge or cloth into the cleaning solution, wring out the excess, and wipe all interior surfaces. For sticky spots, sprinkle a bit of baking soda directly on the area and scrub with a brush.

5. Don't Forget the Door Seals: Use the same solution and a toothbrush to gently scrub the rubber gaskets around the doors—they're often a magnet for crumbs and grime.

6. Rinse and Dry: Wipe all surfaces with a cloth dampened with plain water to remove any leftover cleaning solution. Then dry everything thoroughly with a clean towel or microfiber cloth.

7. Deodorize Naturally: Place an open box of baking soda on a shelf to absorb odors. For a light, natural scent, try adding a few drops of essential oil (like lemon or lavender) to a small bowl of baking soda.

8. Reassemble and Organize: Once everything is clean and dry, return the shelves and drawers, then restock the fridge—putting older food items toward the front to help reduce waste.

Pro Tips:

Using this simple, natural routine, your fridge will stay clean, fresh-smelling, and safer for your food—no chemicals required.

> Wipe down spills as soon as they happen to prevent buildup.
> Deep clean your fridge every 3–6 months.
> Use gentle cloths or sponges to avoid scratching surfaces.

A well-maintained kitchen ensures hygiene and efficiency. By incorporating natural cleaning solutions and regular upkeep, you can keep each kitchen area sparkling clean without the need for harsh chemicals. Consistent cleaning habits will also help prevent costly repairs and extend the lifespan of your appliances and surfaces.

Additional Considerations for the Kitchen

While cleaning and maintaining your kitchen is essential, there are additional factors to consider when ensuring a healthy and pest-free space. From preventing unwanted pests like fruit flies and drain moths to addressing hidden dangers such as fungal growth in sink drains, this chapter explores key concerns and solutions for a cleaner and safer kitchen.

1. Dealing with Fruit Flies

Fruit flies can quickly become a nuisance in any kitchen, especially if fruits and vegetables are left out. These pests lay their eggs in cracks or on overripe produce, leading to rapid infestations.

Preventing Fruit Flies

> Store fruits and vegetables in the refrigerator when possible.
> Regularly take out the trash, especially when disposing of food scraps.
> Clean up spills and crumbs immediately to eliminate food sources.
> Avoid leaving dirty dishes in the sink for extended periods.

Trapping Fruit Flies

One effective way to trap fruit flies is by using a simple homemade trap:

- » Fill a small dish with apple cider vinegar or wine.
- » Add a drop of dish soap to break the surface tension.
- » Cover with plastic wrap and poke small holes to allow flies to enter but not escape.

2. Managing Drain Flies (Moth Flies)

Drain flies, also known as sewer flies or moth flies, are often found near moist, organic-rich areas such as sink drains, garbage disposals, and floor drains. Their larvae feed on the slimy buildup that forms in these areas.

Preventing Drain Fly Infestations

- » Regularly clean sink drains and garbage disposals to remove organic debris.
- » Use a long-handled brush to scrub away buildup in drains.
- » Pour boiling water down the drain once a week to flush out larvae.
- » Avoid pouring bleach down the drain, as it does not effectively remove the slime layer where larvae live.

3. Fungal Growth in Sinks and Drains

Fusarium, a common fungus, has been found in sink drains and can pose potential health risks. Research suggests that these fungi can serve as reservoirs for infections, particularly in individuals with weakened immune systems.[12]

Preventing Fungal Growth

- » Clean and disinfect sink drains regularly with a combination of baking soda and vinegar.
- » Keep the sink dry when not in use to prevent moisture buildup.
- » Use hydrogen peroxide to disinfect and eliminate fungal biofilms.

> Wipe down the sink and surrounding areas to prevent mold spores from spreading.

4. Odor Control in the Kitchen

Kitchen odors can stem from a variety of sources, including garbage disposals, refrigerators, and food spills. Keeping the kitchen smelling fresh requires proactive measures.

Eliminating Odors Naturally

> **Garbage Disposal:** Freeze lemon and vinegar ice cubes and grind them in the disposal to neutralize odors.

> **Refrigerator:** Place an open box of baking soda inside to absorb strong smells. Both charcoal and coffee grounds are also excellent natural solutions for absorbing and neutralizing odors in your refrigerator.

  o **Charcoal:** Place a few pieces of activated charcoal in a breathable container in the back of your refrigerator.

  o **Coffee Grounds:** Spread used coffee grounds on a baking sheet and allow them to dry completely. Once dry, place the grounds in an open container or shallow bowl. Replace the grounds every 2–3 weeks for maximum effectiveness.

> **Trash Cans:** Sprinkle baking soda at the bottom of the trash can before adding a new liner.

> **Microwave:** Heat a bowl of water with lemon slices for a few minutes to loosen grime and freshen the air.

5. Hidden Safety Hazards in the Kitchen

Beyond cleaning, maintaining a safe kitchen environment involves identifying and addressing hidden hazards.

Child Safety Measures

>> Store cleaning products in locked cabinets or out of children's reach.
>> Avoid using chemical-heavy cleaners that may be harmful if ingested.
>> Keep sharp objects like knives and graters securely stored.

Preventing Cross-Contamination

>> Use separate cutting boards for raw meats and vegetables.
>> Wash hands and utensils thoroughly after handling raw food.
>> Sanitize countertops and food prep areas regularly.

A well-maintained kitchen is not only about cleanliness but also about preventing common issues such as pests, fungal growth, and lingering odors. By incorporating simple preventative measures, you can ensure your kitchen remains a safe, hygienic, and pleasant space for cooking and gathering.

Did You Know? Kitchen Ingredients to the Rescue

Cream of Tartar: The Unexpected Hero

Cream of tartar is often found lurking in the back of your spice cabinet, a forgotten friend just waiting to unleash its cleaning potential.

Use it on:

>> **Rust removal (again, because why not?).** Mix cream of tartar with a little water to create a paste, then apply it to rusty metal objects or utensils. Rub it in, rinse, and revel in the rust-free glory.
>> **Whitening your sinks.** You can mix cream of tartar with a little vinegar to scrub your sink and toilet. The abrasive properties help

scrub away grime, leaving your porcelain sparkling like it's auditioning for a role in *The Bachelor*.

> **Fun Fact:** Cream of tartar might sound like something you should bake with, but it's actually a cleaning wizard in disguise. It's like a spice... but for your soul... and your sink.

Ketchup: Your Kitchen's Best Kept Secret

No, you don't need a pricey copper cleaner or tarnish remover. Just reach for that bottle of ketchup you've been neglecting.

Use it on:

> **Copper pots and pans.** Is your copper cookware looking a little too "vintage"? Apply a layer of ketchup, let it sit for 10-15 minutes, then buff away. The acid in the ketchup helps dissolve tarnish, and your pot will shine like new!

> **Stubborn rust stains.** Ketchup is like a sticky little rust-buster. Slather it on rust spots on metal surfaces (like your showerhead or the bottom of your sink), let it work its magic, and scrub it away. No more rust, just a lot of questions about how you discovered this.

> **Fun Fact:** The next time you get ketchup on your clothes, just tell everyone you're testing its cleaning potential. It's all about perspective!

Mayonnaise: The Miracle of Creamy Cleansing

That jar of mayonnaise might have been in your fridge for far too long, but it can also make your life easier when it comes to tackling tough cleaning jobs.

Use it on:

> » **Water rings on wood furniture.** If you've accidentally left a glass of water on your wooden coffee table, don't panic. Apply a small amount of mayonnaise to the water ring, let it sit for 30 minutes, then wipe off with a soft cloth. It works wonders!
>
> » **Sticky residue.** Got old sticker residue or tape marks that just won't budge? Dab a little mayo on the spot, wait for a few minutes, and then wipe away. It's like the sticky stuff is scared of the mayo's creamy dominance.

Fun Fact: Mayonnaise is technically just a combination of eggs and oil, so you might be able to clean and make a sandwich. Efficiency at its finest!

Mustard: The Secret Stain Slayer

You thought mustard was just for hot dogs and burgers? Think again, my friend! Turns out, mustard is a surprising stain-fighting powerhouse.

Use it on:

> » **Grease stains on clothing.** Yes, the mustard stains on your shirt are nothing compared to the stains mustard can erase. Dab mustard onto the greasy mark, let it sit for a few minutes, and then rinse. The enzymes in mustard help break down the oil!
>
> » **Scuff marks on floors.** If your hardwood or linoleum floors have seen better days (we all have that one corner), rub a little mustard on the scuff marks, let it sit, and then wipe it away. It's like magic... or maybe just science. Either way, you're cleaning with mustard.

Fun Fact: If you spill mustard on your floor, no worries—it's practically a cleaning product already!

Tomato Paste: The Sauce That Saves Your Stainless

Tomato paste isn't just for pasta night—it's also a surprisingly powerful partner in crime when it comes to rescuing your burnt, blackened pots.

Use it on:

> **Stainless steel pots with burnt or blackened stains.** Smear a generous amount of tomato paste directly onto the charred areas and let it sit for 20 minutes. The natural acidity in the tomatoes helps break down the burnt bits so you can scrub them away with a walnut or coconut scrub. Rinse, repeat if needed, and boom—your pot is back in business.

> **Bonus Tip:** For really stubborn spots, let the tomato paste hang out a bit longer (up to 30 minutes), but go easy with the scrubbing to avoid scratching that shiny surface.

Fun Fact: Who knew your spaghetti sauce starter could moonlight as a stainless steel stain slayer? Tomato paste isn't just tasty—it's tough.

Vodka: Surprising Uses

Vodka isn't just for cocktails—it can also be a powerful cleaning agent with a variety of household uses:

> **Insect Repellent:** Spray vodka on surfaces to deter insects.

> **Fabric Freshener:** Lightly mist clothing with vodka to neutralize odors between washes.

> **Glass and Chrome Cleaner:** Use vodka on a soft cloth to polish glass, chrome, and porcelain surfaces.

>> **Disinfectant:** The alcohol content makes it an effective natural disinfectant for kitchen surfaces.

>> **Odor Eliminator:** Spray vodka in areas with lingering odors, such as trash cans or cutting boards, to help neutralize smells.

>> **Rust Remover:** No more rust, just a lot of questions from others!

Chapter Notes

1. Su, Y., Xing, B., & Ji, R. (2024). Melamine sponges shed microplastics when scrubbed. ACS Environmental Science & Technology. Retrieved from https://www.acs.org/pressroom/presspacs/2024/june/melamine-sponges-shed-microplastics-when-scrubbed.html

2. Missouri Poison Center. (n.d.). Magic Eraser. Retrieved from https://missouripoisoncenter.org/is-this-a-poison/magic-eraser/

3. Grist. (2015). Are those magic sponges terrible for the environment? Retrieved from https://grist.org/living/are-those-magic-sponges-terrible-for-the-environment/

4. Smithsonian Magazine. (2023). Scientists have created synthetic sponges that soak up microplastics. Retrieved from https://www.smithsonianmag.com/innovation/scientists-have-created-synthetic-sponges-that-soak-up-microplastics-180983017/

5. Environmental Working Group. (2024, September). What are phthalates? https://www.ewg.org/news-insights/news/2024/09/what-are-phthalates

6. Cleveland Clinic. (2022). Triclosan: What it is & effects. https://my.clevelandclinic.org/health/articles/24280-triclosan

7. Medical News Today. (2023). Ammonia in the lungs: Long and short term health implications. https://www.medicalnewstoday.com/articles/ammonia-in-lungs

8. Paloma Health. (2024). Why the chlorine in swimming pools can affect your thyroid. https://www.palomahealth.com/learn/chlorine-swimming-pools-thyroid

9. American Cancer Society. (2024). Formaldehyde and cancer risk. https://www.cancer.org/cancer/risk-prevention/chemicals/formaldehyde.html

10. Agency for Toxic Substances and Disease Registry. (2022). Tetrachloroethylene (PERC) | ToxFAQs™. https://wwwn.cdc.gov/TSP/ToxFAQs/ToxFAQsDetails.aspx?faqid=264&toxid=48

11. Centers for Disease Control and Prevention. (2022). Medical management guidelines for sodium hydroxide (NaOH). https://wwwn.cdc.gov/TSP/MMG/MMGDetails.aspx?mmgid=246&toxid=45

12. Short, D. P. G., O'Donnell, K., Thrane, U., Nielsen, K. F., Zhang, N., Juba, J. H., & Geiser, D. M. (2011). Widespread occurrence of diverse human pathogenic types of the fungus Fusarium detected in plumbing drains. Journal of Clinical Microbiology, 49(11), 4264–4272. https://doi.org/10.1128/JCM.05468-11

CHAPTER 6

Floors & Glass: Sparkling Without Toxins

Introduction: The Hidden Dangers in Common Cleaners

Maintaining clean floors and glass surfaces is essential for a healthy home, but conventional cleaning products often contain harmful chemicals that can pose risks to both human health and the environment.[1] Many of these substances linger on surfaces, get absorbed through the skin, or become airborne, making them hazardous for children, pets, and individuals with respiratory sensitivities.[2] Understanding these risks is the first step toward making safer choices for your household.

Harmful Ingredients in Conventional Floor and Glass Cleaners

Many commercial cleaning products contain a mix of chemicals that can cause irritation, toxicity, or long-term health issues. Below are some of the most concerning ingredients commonly found in floor and glass cleaners.

1. Sodium Lauryl Sulfate (SLS)

> **Purpose:** A surfactant that helps cleaners foam and spread easily.
> **Health Risks:**

- Causes skin irritation and dryness, particularly for sensitive individuals and pets.
- Pets that walk on freshly cleaned floors may ingest SLS by licking their paws, leading to gastrointestinal distress.

- **Scientific Findings:** Studies indicate that prolonged exposure to SLS can negatively impact skin health and may contribute to irritation.[3]

2. Ammonia

» **Purpose:** A powerful grease-cutting agent found in both floor and glass cleaners.

» **Health Risks:**

    o Causes respiratory irritation, coughing, and wheezing, particularly in young children and those with asthma.

    o Toxic when inhaled in large amounts or ingested.

    o Can cause severe irritation to pets' eyes, skin, and respiratory systems.

- **Scientific Findings:** Research suggests that ammonia exposure can worsen asthma and other respiratory conditions.[4]

3. Chlorine Bleach (Sodium Hypochlorite)

» **Purpose:** A disinfectant often used to kill germs and remove stains.

» **Health Risks:**

    o Releases toxic fumes that can irritate the eyes, throat, and lungs.

    o Highly toxic to pets, leading to symptoms such as skin irritation, vomiting, and poisoning if ingested.

» **Scientific Findings:** Studies link bleach exposure to increased respiratory problems in both children and animals.[5]

4. Phthalates

» **Purpose:** Found in scented cleaning products to prolong fragrance.

> **Health Risks:**
>> o Endocrine disruptors that interfere with hormone regulation, affecting reproductive health.
>> o Linked to developmental issues in children and pets.

> **Scientific Findings:** Research associates phthalate exposure with changes in brain development and hormone function.[6]

5. Synthetic Fragrances

> **Purpose:** Added to cleaners to create pleasant scents.
> **Health Risks:**
>> o Can trigger allergic reactions, headaches, and respiratory distress.
>> o Especially harmful to pets, leading to breathing difficulties and skin irritation.

> **Scientific Findings:** Synthetic fragrances have been shown to contribute to indoor air pollution and endocrine disruption.[7]

The Impact on Small Children and Pets

Children and pets are more vulnerable to the effects of toxic cleaning chemicals due to their smaller size and frequent exposure to floors and surfaces.

Small Children:

> More likely to ingest harmful residues by touching floors and putting hands in their mouths.[8]
> Their developing respiratory systems are more susceptible to irritation from airborne chemicals.[9]
> Skin absorption of toxins is higher in young children due to their delicate skin barrier.[10]

Pets:

> ❯ Often lick their paws after walking on cleaned floors, leading to ingestion of toxic residues.

> ❯ Cats, in particular, have difficulty metabolizing certain chemicals, making them highly sensitive to cleaning agents.

> ❯ Birds have delicate respiratory systems and can suffer severe consequences from inhaling chemical fumes.[11]

Reducing Exposure to Harmful Chemicals

To minimize health risks associated with cleaning products, consider adopting safer alternatives:

Read Labels Carefully

> ❯ Avoid products with ammonia, chlorine bleach, SLS, phthalates, and synthetic fragrances.

> ❯ Opt for plant-based, fragrance-free, or organic cleaning solutions.

Improve Ventilation

> ❯ Open windows and doors when using any cleaning product to reduce airborne chemical concentration.

> ❯ Use exhaust fans in areas with poor air circulation.

Use Natural Cleaning Alternatives

> ❯ White vinegar, baking soda, and Castile soap are excellent substitutes that clean effectively without toxic chemicals.

> ❯ Essential oils can be used sparingly for fragrance but should be chosen carefully, as some are harmful to pets.

Switch to Microfiber Cloths

> Microfiber cloths remove dirt and bacteria without the need for chemical cleaners.[12]

Conventional floor and glass cleaners often contain chemicals that can pose serious health risks to both humans and pets. By understanding these risks and making informed choices, you can create a safer, healthier home. Opting for non-toxic alternatives, reading ingredient labels, and improving ventilation are simple yet effective steps toward reducing exposure to harmful substances. A clean home shouldn't come at the cost of your family's health—choosing safer cleaning methods ensures a better environment for everyone.

Healthier Cleaning Alternatives and Found Objects You Can Use for Cleaning Floors and Glass

Switching to non-toxic cleaning alternatives is one of the best ways to protect your home, your health, and the environment. Many household items can be used to clean floors and glass effectively, without exposing your family or pets to harmful chemicals. By utilizing natural ingredients and repurposing common objects, you can achieve a sparkling clean home safely and sustainably.

Healthier Alternatives for Cleaning Floors

1. Vinegar and Water Solution

> **What it is:** A natural disinfectant that removes dirt and grime without harmful residues.

> **How to Use:** Mix ½ cup of white vinegar with 1 gallon of warm water. Mop floors as usual.

>> **Benefits:** Safe for most flooring types, except unsealed wood or stone, where acidity may cause damage.

2. Baking Soda Paste

>> **What it is:** A mild abrasive that helps scrub away stains and grime.

>> **How to Use:** Sprinkle baking soda directly on the floor and scrub gently with a damp cloth or mop.

>> **Benefits:** Neutralizes odors and cleans without toxic fumes. Beware of using baking soda on hardwood floors however, because it can damage the finish over time.

3. Castile Soap Solution

>> **What it is:** A plant-based, biodegradable soap safe for all surfaces.

>> **How to Use:** Mix 1-2 tablespoons of Castile soap with a gallon of warm water. Mop floors as usual.

>> **Benefits:** Effective at cutting grease and safe for children and pets.

Healthier Alternatives for Cleaning Glass

1. Vinegar and Water Spray

>> **What it is:** A natural degreaser and disinfectant.

>> **How to Use:** Mix equal parts white vinegar and water in a spray bottle. Spray on glass surfaces and wipe with a microfiber cloth.

>> **Benefits:** Leaves a streak-free shine without chemical residues.

2. Witch Hazel Solution

>> **What it is:** A natural astringent that cleans without leaving streaks.

>> **How to Use:** Mix ¼ cup witch hazel, ¼ cup water, and ¼ cup vinegar in a spray bottle. Wipe with a microfiber cloth or newspaper.

>> **Benefits:** Dissolves grime and dries quickly, reducing smudges.

3. Cornstarch Glass Cleaner

- **What it is:** An alternative ingredient that enhances shine.
- **How to Use:** Mix 1 tablespoon cornstarch with ½ cup white vinegar and ½ cup water in a spray bottle. Shake well and apply to glass surfaces.
- **Benefits:** Reduces streaking and provides a polished finish.

Found Objects for Cleaning Floors and Glass

1. Microfiber Cloths

- **How to Use:** Damp microfiber cloths trap dust and dirt without chemicals.
- **Benefits:** Reusable and highly effective at removing residue from floors and glass.

2. Old T-Shirts or Towels

- **How to Use:** Cut into rags for scrubbing floors or polishing glass.
- **Benefits:** Reduces waste and repurposes old fabrics.

3. Newspapers

- **How to Use:** Use crumpled newspapers to wipe glass after applying cleaner.
- **Benefits:** Leaves glass streak-free without lint.

4. Toothbrushes

- **How to Use:** Use an old toothbrush to scrub grout and tight corners.
- **Benefits:** Reaches small areas that mops and sponges can't clean.

5. Coffee Filters

> **How to Use:** Spray your mirror or glass with a vinegar-water solution, then wipe with a clean coffee filter in circular motions for a streak-free finish.

> **Benefits:** Lint-free, absorbent, and a budget-friendly alternative to paper towels—perfect for crystal-clear glass without waste.

Switching to natural cleaning alternatives and repurposing household items can make cleaning safer, more effective, and eco-friendly. Simple solutions like vinegar and witch hazel eliminate the need for toxic chemicals, while reusable cloths and household tools reduce waste. By making mindful choices, you can create a healthier home for your family and pets while protecting the environment.

How to and Recipes for Cleaning Floors and Glass

Creating your own cleaning solutions ensures that your home stays free from harmful chemicals while still maintaining spotless floors and crystal-clear glass surfaces. These simple, effective recipes use natural ingredients that are safe for children, pets, and the environment.

How to Clean Floors Naturally

1. Basic Vinegar Floor Cleaner

> **Ingredients:**
>   - ½ cup white vinegar
>   - 1 gallon warm water

> **Instructions:**
>   - Mix the vinegar and water in a bucket.
>   - Mop floors as usual, ensuring excess liquid is wrung out to prevent streaking.

> **Best For:** Tile, laminate, and vinyl flooring.
> **Note:** Avoid using vinegar on unsealed wood or natural stone, as it may cause damage.

2. Baking Soda Scrub for Tough Stains

> **Ingredients:**
>   o   2 tablespoons baking soda
>   o   1 cup warm water

> **Instructions:**
>   o   Apply the paste to stubborn stains.
>   o   Scrub with a soft brush or cloth.
>   o   Rinse with water and dry with a towel.

> **Best For:** Removing sticky residues and scuffs on hard floors like tile. Beware of use on hardwood floors because it can damage the finish over time.

3. Castile Soap Gentle Floor Wash

> **Ingredients:**
>   o   1-2 tablespoons liquid Castile soap
>   o   1 gallon warm water

> **Instructions:**
>   o   Mix the soap and water in a bucket.
>   o   Mop floors as usual.

> **Best For:** Hardwood and sealed stone floors.

How to Clean Glass Surfaces Naturally

1. Streak-Free Vinegar Glass Cleaner

- **Ingredients:**
  - 1 cup white vinegar
  - 1 cup water
  - 1 tablespoon rubbing alcohol (optional, for extra shine)
- **Instructions:**
  - Combine ingredients in a spray bottle and shake well.
  - Spray onto glass and wipe with a microfiber cloth or newspaper.
- **Best For:** Windows, mirrors, and glass tabletops.

2. Witch Hazel and Cornstarch Glass Cleaner

- **Ingredients:**
  - ¼ cup witch hazel
  - ¼ cup white vinegar
  - 1 tablespoon cornstarch
  - ½ cup water
- **Instructions:**
  - Shake ingredients together in a spray bottle.
  - Spray onto glass and wipe with a lint-free cloth.
- **Best For:** Reducing streaks and enhancing shine on all glass surfaces.

3. Lemon Juice and Water Polish

- **Ingredients:**
  - 2 tablespoons lemon juice
  - 1 cup water
- **Instructions:**
  - Mix in a spray bottle.
  - Spray onto glass and wipe with a clean cloth.
- **Best For:** Adding a fresh scent while removing grime.

Tips for Effective Natural Cleaning

> **Use Microfiber Cloths:** They trap dirt and dust without the need for chemical sprays.
> **Polish with Newspapers:** A great eco-friendly way to get streak-free glass.
> **Avoid Excess Liquid on Wood Floors:** Too much moisture can cause damage, so always wring out mops thoroughly.
> **Label DIY Cleaners:** Store homemade solutions in clearly labeled spray bottles to prevent confusion.

Homemade cleaning solutions using simple ingredients like vinegar, baking soda, Castile soap, and essential oils are highly effective, safe, and affordable. By making your own cleaners, you can maintain a spotless home while keeping harmful chemicals out of your living space. Enjoy the benefits of a cleaner, healthier home with these natural cleaning recipes!

Additional Considerations

Beyond Basic Cleaning for Floors and Glass

While choosing non-toxic cleaning solutions is a crucial step, there are additional factors to consider when maintaining floors and glass surfaces. Proper care and maintenance can extend the lifespan of your floors and glass while ensuring they remain safe and free of harmful residues. This section explores key considerations such as avoiding residue buildup, preventing damage, and maintaining the longevity of your surfaces.

Preventing Residue Buildup on Floors and Glass

1. Rinsing and Drying Floors Properly

» Even natural cleaners can leave residue if not rinsed properly.

» Always use a damp (not soaking wet) mop to remove excess cleaning solution.

» Dry floors with a clean microfiber cloth to prevent streaking and water damage.

2. Avoiding Soap Scum on Glass Surfaces

» Soap-based cleaners can leave a cloudy film on glass surfaces.

» Use a vinegar-water solution or rubbing alcohol to break down buildup.

» Wipe glass with a lint-free microfiber cloth or newspaper for a streak-free finish.

Protecting Floors from Damage

1. Choosing the Right Cleaning Tools

» Use soft-bristle brooms or microfiber mops to avoid scratching floors.

» Avoid using abrasive sponges or steel wool on any flooring surface.

» For glass surfaces, use non-abrasive cloths to prevent scratches and smudges.

2. Preventing Water Damage

» Excessive moisture can warp wood and cause damage to laminate floors.

» Always wring out mops before use and never allow water to pool on the surface.

» For glass, avoid using excessive liquid, especially near window edges where it can seep into frames.

3. Using Floor Mats and Protective Pads

> Place doormats at entrances to reduce dirt and debris brought inside.
> Use felt pads under furniture legs to prevent scratches on hard flooring.
> Avoid wearing high heels or dragging heavy furniture across floors to prevent dents and scuffs.

Maintaining the Longevity of Floors and Glass

1. Regular Maintenance for Floors

> Sweep or vacuum floors daily to remove dust and prevent buildup.
> Use a gentle cleaner once a week to maintain a clean surface without over washing.
> Reapply a protective finish (if applicable) to wooden floors periodically.

2. Keeping Glass Crystal Clear

> Clean glass at least once a week to prevent grime buildup.
> Avoid cleaning windows on hot, sunny days, as this can cause streaking.
> Use a squeegee for large glass surfaces to achieve a professional finish.

The Steam Cleaning Controversy: Pros, Cons, and Considerations

Steam cleaning has gained popularity as an effective and eco-friendly method for sanitizing floors without harsh chemicals. However, its use—particularly on hardwood floors—has sparked debate among homeowners and cleaning experts.

Why Is Steam Cleaning Controversial?

The controversy largely centers around the potential risks steam poses to certain flooring types, especially hardwood. While steam cleaning offers impressive sanitization by killing bacteria and loosening grime with high heat, it also carries inherent dangers for moisture-sensitive surfaces.

Potential Risks for Hardwood Floors

Hardwood floors are particularly vulnerable to steam cleaning due to the combination of heat and moisture. Even though most steam mops claim to produce "dry" steam, moisture can still penetrate cracks, joints, and gaps in the wood. Over time, this can lead to:

> **Moisture Damage:** The absorbed moisture may cause hardwood planks to swell, warp, or buckle. This is especially true for older floors or those with imperfect seals.

> **Warranty Voiding:** Many hardwood floor manufacturers explicitly state that steam cleaning voids their product warranty. This is because steam cleaning is considered an aggressive cleaning method that can compromise the protective finish.

> **Discoloration:** Excess moisture may cause fading, dulling, or dark spots on hardwood floors, especially if the finish is already worn or damaged.

Safer Alternatives and Best Practices

While some homeowners successfully use steam mops on sealed hardwood with no immediate issues, it's crucial to follow best practices to minimize risk:

> **Test in a Small Area:** Always start by testing your steam cleaner on an inconspicuous area to assess its impact.

> **Use Low Heat Settings:** Some steam mops offer adjustable temperature settings; choosing a lower setting reduces the risk of excessive heat exposure.

> **Avoid Lingering in One Spot:** Keeping the mop in motion prevents excess moisture buildup in any one area.

> **Check Manufacturer Guidelines:** Always review your flooring manufacturer's care instructions to avoid inadvertently voiding the warranty.

The Debate on Tile and Vinyl Floors

While tile and vinyl floors are generally considered safer for steam cleaning, there are still concerns. Steam may weaken adhesives in vinyl flooring over time or cause grout in tile floors to degrade if not properly sealed.

Maintaining clean and well-preserved floors and glass surfaces requires more than just choosing the right cleaners—it also involves proper techniques and preventive measures. By using the right tools, preventing residue buildup, and protecting surfaces from damage, you can ensure the longevity and appearance of your floors and glass while keeping them free from harmful chemicals. Implementing these additional considerations will help create a safe, beautiful, and well-maintained home environment.

Did You Know? Surprising Recipes and Tips for Cleaner Floors

Glass and All Purpose Cleaning Recipes

Glass cleaner:

> 1 cup hot water
> ½ tbsp. cornstarch
> ⅛ cup vinegar

>> ⅛ cup rubbing alcohol

Streak free outside window cleaner:

>> 2 tbsp. Dawn
>> 2 cups vinegar
>> 2 gal. hot water
>> Foam squeegee

Instructions: Remove screens, spray down windows with water first. Clean windows using a foam squeegee with solution, then let air dry.

All Purpose cleaner:

>> 1 cup water
>> Orange peels
>> 1 cup vinegar
>> ¼ cup lemon juice

Instructions: Start with the water first, then add the orange peels. Let sit for 1-2 minutes. Add vinegar and add the lemon juice all in a spray bottle.

Tips for Cleaner Laminate Floors

Dry mop laminate floors first starting from the edges and creating a pile of dirt. Vacuum. Damp mop with a solution mixed with Dawn soap and warm water. Mop with a saturated, clean microfiber mop going with the grain of the wood.

Chapter Notes

1. Environmental Working Group. (2023, September). Cleaning products emit hundreds of hazardous chemicals, new study finds. https://www.ewg.org/news-insights/news-release/2023/09/cleaning-products-emit-hundreds-hazardous-chemicals-new-study

2. California Air Resources Board. (n.d.). Cleaning products and indoor air quality. https://ww2.arb.ca.gov/resources/fact-sheets/cleaning-products-indoor-air-quality

3. Wilhelm, K. P., Surber, C., & Maibach, H. I. (1991). Effect of sodium lauryl sulfate-induced skin irritation on in vitro percutaneous absorption of four drugs. Journal of Investigative Dermatology, 96(1), 125–129. https://doi.org/10.1111/1523-1747.ep12357745

4. U.S. Environmental Protection Agency. (2016). Toxicological review of ammonia (noncancer inhalation). https://iris.epa.gov/static/pdfs/0422_summary.pdf

5. Centers for Disease Control and Prevention. (n.d.). Public health statement for chlorine. https://wwwn.cdc.gov/TSP/PHS/PHS.aspx?phsid=683&toxid=36

6. Benjamin, S., Masai, E., Kamimura, N., Takahashi, K., Anderson, R. C., & Faisal, P. A. (2017). Phthalates impact human health: Epidemiological evidences and plausible mechanism of action. Journal of Hazardous Materials, 340, 360–383. https://doi.org/10.1016/j.jhazmat.2017.06.036

7. Steinemann, A. (2016). Fragranced consumer products: Exposures and effects from emissions. Air Quality, Atmosphere & Health, 9(3), 275–281. https://doi.org/10.1007/s11869-016-0442-z

8. U.S. Environmental Protection Agency. (n.d.). Understanding exposures in children's environments. https://www.epa.gov/healthresearch/understanding-exposures-childrens-environments

9. World Health Organization. (2011). Children and chemicals. https://apps.who.int/iris/bitstream/handle/10665/370534/WHO-FWC-PHE-EPE-11.01-eng.pdf

10. U.S. Environmental Protection Agency. (n.d.). Understanding exposures in children's environments. https://www.epa.gov/healthresearch/understanding-exposures-childrens-environments

11. The Nature of Home. (2024, December 15). Protect your pet: 18 hidden dangers in common cleaners. https://thenatureofhome.com/protect-your-pet-18-hidden-dangers-in-common-cleaners/

12. GreenyPlace. (n.d.). Does microfiber really remove bacteria? Retrieved from https://greenyplace.com/does-microfiber-really-remove-bacteria

CHAPTER 7

Laundry Room: Fresh Clothes, No Toxins

Avoiding Harmful Chemicals in the Laundry Room

The laundry room is often overlooked as a source of harmful chemicals in the home. Many conventional laundry products contain ingredients that may contribute to indoor air pollution, skin irritation, and environmental harm.[1,2] Understanding what's in these products and how to replace them with safer alternatives is essential for a healthier home and planet.

The Hidden Dangers in Common Laundry Products

Dryer Sheets: A Chemical Concern

Dryer sheets are a staple in many households, but their safety is questionable. These sheets are coated with chemical fabric softeners that reduce static cling and impart a soft feel to clothing. However, research indicates that these chemicals may release harmful volatile organic compounds (VOCs) into the air.

A 2010 study from the University of Washington analyzed 25 popular fragranced consumer products, including laundry detergents, fabric softeners, and dryer sheets. The study found that each product emitted at least one chemical classified as toxic or hazardous under federal laws. Some VOCs detected in dryer sheets are classified as carcinogens with no safe exposure level, according to the U.S. Environmental Protection Agency.[3]

A follow-up study in 2011 further examined the issue, revealing that dryer vents release hazardous chemicals into the air.[4] Unlike emissions from vehicles and industrial sources, these chemicals are unregulated and unmonitored. Given this evidence, it is advisable to avoid fragranced dryer sheets altogether and seek safer alternatives.

Fabric Softeners: The Hidden Risks

Liquid fabric softeners work by coating fabric fibers with a thin layer of chemicals that reduce static cling and impart a silky texture. While they may seem harmless, many contain artificial fragrances and chemicals that can irritate the skin and respiratory system.[5]

Fabric softeners are cationic, meaning they bind to negatively charged fabric fibers. However, this binding process involves synthetic compounds that can leave behind residues harmful to people with sensitive skin or allergies. Moreover, the fragrance mixtures used in fabric softeners are often undisclosed, making it impossible to know what chemicals are being inhaled or absorbed through the skin.[6]

Laundry Detergents: Toxic Ingredients to Avoid

Conventional laundry detergents often contain surfactants, optical brighteners, and artificial fragrances that can be harsh on both skin and the environment. Some common harmful ingredients include:

> **Sodium Lauryl Sulfate (SLS) and Sodium Laureth Sulfate (SLES):** These surfactants create foaming action but can cause skin irritation.[7]
> **Phosphates:** These contribute to water pollution, leading to harmful algal blooms that deplete oxygen in aquatic ecosystems.[8]
> **Chlorine Bleach:** A strong disinfectant that emits toxic fumes and can be irritating to the skin and lungs.[9]

> **Optical Brighteners:** Chemicals that make clothes appear brighter but do not actually clean; they can cause skin irritation and may be toxic to aquatic life.[10]

By eliminating harmful chemicals from your laundry routine, you create a healthier living environment and reduce your ecological footprint.

Healthier Laundry Alternatives

Switching to healthier laundry alternatives can greatly reduce exposure to harmful chemicals while also being more environmentally friendly. Here are some natural and effective ways to keep your laundry fresh and clean without compromising on health.

Natural Laundry Detergents

Castile Soap: A Gentle Laundry Detergent

Castile soap, a plant-based soap made from olive oil or coconut oil, can be used as a mild yet effective laundry detergent. It is especially beneficial for those with sensitive skin or allergies.

Simple Castile Soap Laundry Detergent Recipe:

> ¼ cup liquid Castile soap

> ¼ cup baking soda (optional, for stain removal)

> 1 tablespoon white vinegar (optional, for softening fabrics)

To use, add the Castile soap directly into the detergent compartment or the drum of the washing machine. If using baking soda, sprinkle it into the drum before starting the wash cycle.

Borax and Washing Soda: A Powerful Laundry Detergent Alternative

Borax and washing soda are natural, affordable, and effective alternatives to traditional laundry detergents. Both are known for their powerful cleaning abilities, helping to break down stains, neutralize odors, and soften hard water.[11, 12]

Simple Borax and Washing Soda Laundry Detergent Recipe:

> ½ cup borax
> ½ cup washing soda
> ¼ cup grated soap (Castile soap or any natural bar soap)

To use, mix the ingredients thoroughly and store in an airtight container. For each load of laundry, add 2 tablespoons of the detergent directly into the drum before starting the wash cycle. For extra cleaning power or stubborn stains, add an additional tablespoon of washing soda to the load.

Other Considerations for a Healthier Laundry Routine

> **Wash with Cold Water:** Reduces energy consumption and helps preserve fabrics.
> **Use Fragrance-Free and Eco-Friendly Detergents:** Many brands offer plant-based, biodegradable detergents free from synthetic fragrances and dyes.
> **Air Dry When Possible:** Line drying clothes reduces energy use and extends the life of garments.

Soap Nuts: A Plant-Based Alternative

Soap nuts, also known as soapberries, contain natural saponins that act as a mild detergent. They are completely biodegradable, making them an excellent zero-waste option.[13] They can be found at various stores and online retailers. Common places to purchase them include health food stores like Whole Foods, Amazon, and natural and eco-friendly retailers.

How to Use Soap Nuts:

1. Place 4-5 soap nuts in a small muslin bag.
2. Add the bag to the washing machine drum.
3. Use warm water for best results.
4. Reuse the soap nuts for 4-5 washes before composting them.

Fabric Softening Alternatives

White Vinegar as a Fabric Softener

White vinegar naturally softens fabrics, reduces odors, and breaks down detergent residue. It is a great alternative to chemical-based fabric softeners.

How to Use:

1. Add ¼ to ½ cup of white vinegar to the fabric softener compartment of your washing machine.
2. For added freshness, mix in a few drops of essential oil.

Baking Soda for Freshness

Baking soda neutralizes odors and softens fabrics without the need for artificial fragrances.

How to Use:

1. Add ¼ cup of baking soda to the drum before washing.
2. Works especially well for towels and gym clothes.

Dryer Alternatives

Wool Dryer Balls: A Sustainable Option

Wool dryer balls are a fantastic alternative to dryer sheets. They help reduce drying time, soften clothes, and minimize static.

How to Use Wool Dryer Balls:

1. Use 2-4 balls for small loads, 5-7 balls for large loads.
2. Add a few drops of essential oil for a natural fragrance.
3. Dryer balls last for months, making them a cost-effective solution.

Stain Removal with Natural Ingredients

Lemon Juice for Whites

Lemon juice acts as a natural bleach, helping to brighten white clothes.

How to Use:

1. Add ¼ cup of lemon juice to the wash cycle.
2. Let clothes dry in the sun for an extra whitening boost.

Hydrogen Peroxide for Tough Stains

Hydrogen peroxide is a non-toxic alternative to chlorine bleach, effective for removing stains.

How to Use:

1. Apply 3% hydrogen peroxide directly to stains.
2. Let it sit for 5-10 minutes before washing as usual.

Additional Laundry Tips

> **Wash with Cold Water:** Helps preserve fabrics and reduce energy consumption.

> **Use a Microplastic Filter:** Captures synthetic fibers that shed during washing, preventing water pollution.

> **Line Dry When Possible:** Air drying clothes extends their lifespan and eliminates the need for artificial fabric softeners.

Switching to healthier laundry alternatives benefits both your household and the environment. By choosing plant-based detergents, natural fabric softeners, and sustainable drying methods, you can enjoy fresh, clean laundry without exposure to unnecessary chemicals. Small changes in your laundry routine can make a significant impact on your health and sustainability efforts.

Safely Cleaning Your Washer and Dryer

Maintaining a clean washer and dryer is essential for ensuring that your laundry stays fresh, hygienic, and free from unwanted residues. Over time, detergent buildup, mold, and lint accumulation can impact both the effectiveness and safety of your appliances. Here's how to naturally and effectively clean your washer and dryer using safe, eco-friendly methods.

Cleaning Your Washer

Front-Loading vs. Top-Loading Machines

Both front-loading and top-loading washing machines require regular cleaning to prevent mold, mildew, and soap scum buildup. While front-loaders are more prone to mold due to their rubber gasket, top-loaders can accumulate detergent residues in the drum and dispensers.

Natural Cleaning Solution for Your Washer

What You Need:

1. 2 cups white vinegar (natural disinfectant and deodorizer)
2. ½ cup baking soda (removes odors and detergent buildup)
3. A few drops of tea tree or lavender essential oil (optional for additional antibacterial properties)

How to Clean Your Washer:

1. **Run a Hot Water Cycle with Vinegar:** Pour 2 cups of white vinegar into the detergent dispenser and run the machine on the hottest, longest cycle.
2. **Add Baking Soda:** Once the cycle finishes, sprinkle ½ cup of baking soda into the drum and run another hot water cycle.
3. **Wipe Down the Gasket & Drum:** For front-loaders, thoroughly clean the rubber gasket with a mixture of vinegar and water using a microfiber cloth.
4. **Leave the Door Open:** After every wash, keep the washer door slightly open to allow air circulation and prevent mold growth.

Deep Cleaning the Detergent Dispenser & Filters

- Remove and soak the detergent dispenser in a solution of hot water and vinegar for 15-20 minutes.
- Use a small brush or an old toothbrush to scrub away any detergent buildup.
- For top-loaders, check and clean the fabric softener dispenser and lint trap (if applicable).

Cleaning Your Dryer

Removing Lint Buildup

Lint buildup in the dryer can reduce efficiency and pose a fire hazard. Regularly removing lint from the filter and vents helps keep your dryer running safely.

Steps to Clean the Lint Trap:

1. Remove lint after every load to ensure proper airflow.
2. Wash the lint filter monthly with warm soapy water to remove fabric softener residue.
3. Use a vacuum attachment to clean any trapped lint in the filter housing.

Deep Cleaning the Dryer Vent

Dryer vents can accumulate a significant amount of lint over time, reducing efficiency and increasing fire risks.

How to Clean the Dryer Vent:

1. Unplug the dryer and pull it away from the wall.
2. Disconnect the vent hose and vacuum out any lint buildup inside.
3. Use a vent brush to remove debris from the duct.
4. Reconnect the vent and ensure it is not crushed or kinked, which can restrict airflow.

Deodorizing and Disinfecting the Drum

Just like washing machines, dryer drums can harbor bacteria and residue from fabric softeners and dryer sheets.

What You Need:

> ½ cup white vinegar

- » A damp cloth or sponge
- » A few drops of lemon essential oil (optional)

How to Clean the Dryer Drum:

1. Dampen a cloth with white vinegar and wipe down the inside of the drum.
2. For stubborn stains or odors, mix vinegar with baking soda and scrub lightly.
3. Allow the dryer to air out before the next use.

Additional Dryer Maintenance Tips

- Check and tighten any loose hoses or connections to prevent leaks or inefficiencies.
- Ensure proper ventilation by keeping the exhaust vent free from blockages.
- Avoid overloading the dryer, as this can increase drying time and wear on the motor.

Regularly cleaning your washer and dryer with natural ingredients like vinegar and baking soda keeps your appliances functioning efficiently while eliminating harmful residues. Safe maintenance practices prevent mold, mildew, and fire hazards, ensuring a healthier and more sustainable laundry routine. Taking a few simple steps to clean your appliances can significantly improve their lifespan and performance while keeping your home free from unnecessary toxins.

Additional Considerations

While choosing natural cleaning methods and safer laundry products is a significant step toward a healthier home, there are additional considerations to enhance your eco-friendly laundry routine. These factors can help you reduce environmental impact, save energy, and improve the longevity of your clothing and appliances.

Energy-Efficient Laundry Practices

Wash with Cold Water

Washing clothes in cold water reduces energy consumption, lowers utility bills, and helps preserve fabric quality. Most modern detergents are designed to work efficiently in cold water, ensuring effective cleaning while reducing the carbon footprint of your laundry routine.

Use the Right Load Size

Overloading the washing machine can reduce cleaning effectiveness, while underloading wastes water and energy. Aim for full but not overcrowded loads to optimize efficiency.

Air Dry Whenever Possible

Line drying or using a drying rack instead of a tumble dryer helps extend the lifespan of clothes and reduces energy consumption. If using a dryer, choosing the lowest effective heat setting can also help protect fabrics while saving energy.

Choosing Sustainable Laundry Products

Look for Eco-Friendly Certifications

When purchasing laundry detergents, stain removers, or fabric softeners, look for certifications such as:

> » **EPA Safer Choice** – Ensures products contain safer ingredients.

> **USDA Certified Biobased** – Indicates plant-based content and lower reliance on petroleum-based ingredients.
> **ECOLOGO or EWG Verified** – Ensures environmental and health safety standards.

Avoid Microplastics in Detergents

Some commercial detergents contain synthetic polymers that contribute to microplastic pollution. Opt for natural, biodegradable detergents to minimize environmental impact.

Use Refillable or Plastic-Free Packaging

Reducing plastic waste is another way to make your laundry routine more sustainable. Consider refill stations, cardboard detergent boxes, or reusable glass containers.

Protecting Clothing and Reducing Waste

Wash Less Frequently

Not all clothes need to be washed after every wear. Jeans, sweaters, and jackets can often be worn multiple times before laundering. Spot cleaning and airing out garments can help maintain their freshness while conserving water and energy.

Use a Guppyfriend Bag or Microfiber Filter

Synthetic fabrics shed microfibers during washing, which end up in waterways and harm marine life. Using a Guppyfriend washing bag or installing a microfiber filter in your machine can help trap these particles and prevent pollution.

Repair Instead of Replace

Extending the life of your clothes through minor repairs, such as sewing buttons, fixing small tears, or reinforcing seams, helps reduce textile waste and minimizes the environmental impact of clothing production.

Reducing Allergens and Irritants

Fragrance-Free and Hypoallergenic Options

Many people experience skin irritation due to artificial fragrances in laundry products. Opting for fragrance-free or hypoallergenic detergents, or using natural scent boosters like essential oils, can help reduce allergic reactions and respiratory issues.

Avoid Optical Brighteners and Dyes

These additives make clothes appear whiter and brighter but don't actually enhance cleaning. They can leave behind residues that may cause skin irritation and are often not biodegradable.

Making informed choices about your laundry routine helps promote a healthier home environment, reduces environmental impact, and extends the lifespan of clothing and appliances. From energy-efficient practices and eco-friendly products to waste reduction strategies, small changes can have a significant impact. By adopting these additional considerations, you ensure that your laundry routine aligns with a sustainable and health-conscious lifestyle.

Did You Know? Fresh Clothes and Moth Balls Beware

Cedar Blocks and Charcoal

Cedar blocks and charcoal are natural, effective solutions for keeping clothing fresh, dry, and protected in storage. Each offers distinct benefits, and they can even be used together for optimal results.

Cedar blocks naturally repel moths, absorb moisture, and leave a fresh scent. Use in drawers, closets, or bins. Refresh by sanding every 6–12 months. Charcoal absorbs odors and moisture, preventing mold. Use activated charcoal bags in storage areas and refresh in sunlight every few months.

Best Practice: Combine both for maximum protection—cedar for pests and scent, charcoal for moisture and odor control. Ensure clothes are clean and dry before storing.

Natural Enzymes

Enzyme Power in Action: Did you know you can create your own enzyme cleaner using just citrus peels, sugar, and water? The fermentation process creates natural enzymes and alcohol that break down dirt, grease, and stains.

How It Works:

> **Step 1:** Combine 10 parts warm water, 3 parts citrus peels, and 1 part sugar in a tightly sealed bottle (like a soda bottle).
> **Step 2:** Shake well, then store the bottle in a warm spot.
> **Step 3:** For the first week, loosen the cap daily to release built-up gas. After that, release the pressure every other day for a few weeks, then weekly until it's ready.

> **Step 4:** After 3 months, strain the liquid — your enzyme cleaner is ready to use!

Why It Works: During fermentation, yeast naturally breaks down the sugar into alcohol, which acts as a solvent to dissolve stains. Citrus peels contribute enzymes that help break down grease, protein, and organic matter.

Troubleshooting Tips:

> **Gas Buildup:** Don't forget to "burp" your container to release pressure. Soda bottles are ideal because they can handle the expanding gas.

> **Mold Woes:** If you see white mold, add a little more sugar to restart fermentation and push out unwanted bacteria.

> **Vinegar Smell:** Too much oxygen in the bottle can create a vinegary odor — it's still safe to use, but adding a few drops of citrus essential oil can help improve the scent.

Citrus Peels — Not Just for Snacks: After straining, those leftover peels can still be put to good use! Try adding them to compost, using them to scrub sinks, or tossing them into your garbage disposal for a fresh scent.

Shake It Up: When starting your enzyme cleaner, shake the container well — dancing while you do it is optional, but highly encouraged!

The Danger of Mothballs

Mothballs contain chemicals like naphthalene or paradichlorobenzene, which release toxic fumes that kill moths and other insects. These fumes can pose serious health risks to humans and pets if inhaled, ingested, or if prolonged exposure occurs. Symptoms of exposure may include headaches, dizziness, nausea, and respiratory irritation. Long-term exposure can harm the liver, kidneys, and nervous system, and naphthalene is classified as a possible human carcinogen.[14, 15]

Mothballs are particularly dangerous to children and pets, who may mistake them for candy.[16] Accidental ingestion can cause serious poisoning, including anemia, organ damage, or even death in severe cases.[17] For safer alternatives, consider cedar blocks or activated charcoal for pest control in clothing storage.

Chapter Notes

1. Steinemann, A. (2011, August 24). Scented laundry products emit hazardous chemicals through dryer vents. University of Washington News. https://www.washington.edu/news/2011/08/24/scented-laundry-products-emit-hazardous-chemicals-through-dryer-vents/

2. Unsustainable Magazine. (2023, August 15). The Health and Environmental Impacts of Laundry Practices. https://www.unsustainablemagazine.com/environmental-impacts-of-laundry/

3. Steinemann, A. (2011). Chemical emissions from residential dryer vents during use of fragranced laundry products. Environmental Health Perspectives, 119(7), 944–949. https://doi.org/10.1289/ehp.1103413

4. Steinemann, A. (2011). Dryer vents: An overlooked source of pollution? Environmental Health Perspectives, 119(7), A300–A301. https://doi.org/10.1289/ehp.119-a300

5. Environmental Working Group. (2022, August 15). Skip the most toxic fabric softeners. https://www.ewg.org/news-insights/news/2022/08/skip-most-toxic-fabric-softeners

6. Mullans, E. (n.d.). Here's Why Fabric Softener is Bad News For You and Your Washing. Uptown Dermatology. https://www.uptowndermatologyhouston.com/blog-news/heres-why-fabric-softener-is-bad

7. Hibino, T., & Nishiyama, T. (2015). Quantification of sodium lauryl sulfate penetration into the skin and its effect on skin barrier function. Journal of Dermatological Science, 80(3), 180–186. https://doi.org/10.1016/j.jdermsci.2015.08.009

8. Wang, Y., et al. (2021). Mitigating phosphorus pollution from detergents in the surface waters of China. Science of The Total Environment, 777, 146033. https://doi.org/10.1016/j.scitotenv.2021.146033

9. Centers for Disease Control and Prevention. (2019). Medical Management Guidelines for Chlorine. https://wwwn.cdc.gov/TSP/MMG/MMGDetails.aspx?mmgid=198&toxid=36

10. Dirty Labs. (n.d.). Ask Dr. Pete: What are Optical Brighteners and Why Should We Care? https://dirtylabs.com/blogs/the-dirt/what-are-optical-brighteners-and-why-should-you-care

11. U.S. Borax. (n.d.). Uses of borax for laundry. Retrieved May 15, 2025, from https://www.borax.com/news-events/april-2021/uses-of-borax-for-laundry

12. The Spruce. (2021, November 18). What is washing soda? Retrieved from https://www.thespruce.com/what-is-washing-soda-2145888

13. Greenify Me. (2022, September 1). How to use soap nuts. Retrieved May 15, 2025, from https://www.greenify-me.com/2022/09/how-to-use-soap-nuts.html

14. National Pesticide Information Center. (n.d.). Naphthalene fact sheet. Oregon State University. Retrieved May 15, 2025, from https://npic.orst.edu/factsheets/naphgen.html

15. National Pesticide Information Center. (n.d.). Paradichlorobenzene fact sheet. Oregon State University. Retrieved May 15, 2025, from https://npic.orst.edu/factsheets/PDBgen.html

16. UConn Health. (n.d.). Mothballs can be dangerous to children. Connecticut Poison Control Center. Retrieved May 15, 2025, from https://health.uconn.edu/poison-control/wp-content/uploads/sites/76/2016/12/tipsheet_mothballs.pdf

17. Pet Poison Helpline. (n.d.). Mothballs are toxic to dogs. Retrieved May 15, 2025, from https://www.petpoisonhelpline.com/poison/mothballs/

CHAPTER 8

Dust & Air: Creating a Healthier Home Environment

What You Need to Know About Dust, Air Quality, and Allergens

Understanding Indoor Air Quality

Indoor air quality is a critical aspect of maintaining a healthy home environment. Many factors contribute to indoor air pollution, including biological pollutants, inadequate ventilation, and environmental contaminants. Understanding these factors can help you take steps to improve air quality and protect your health.

Biological Pollutants and Their Effects

Biological pollutants include molds, bacteria, viruses, pollen, animal dander, and particles from dust mites. These can cause infections, provoke allergic reactions, and trigger asthma attacks. The best way to control these pollutants is through regular cleaning, washing bedding to kill dust mites, and controlling moisture levels to prevent mold growth.[1]

The Impact of Poor Air Quality on Health

Exposure to poor indoor air quality can lead to several health issues, such as:

> Respiratory problems, including aggravated asthma and infections
> Headaches, fatigue, and nausea
> Skin and eye irritation

> Neurotoxic symptoms in some individuals. Neurotoxic symptoms can be wide ranging, but include things like difficulty concentrating or mental fog, muscle weakness, burning sensations, dizziness or fainting, and more. A full list can be found on the CDC website.[2]

Symptoms vary based on individual sensitivity and may resemble those of colds or other viral infections, making it difficult to pinpoint air quality as the cause. If symptoms fade when you are away from home and return when you come back, it may indicate an air quality problem.[3]

Common Signs of Poor Air Quality

Indicators of poor air quality include:

> Condensation on windows or walls
> Stale, stuffy air
> Mold growth on books, shoes, or other household items
> Unpleasant odors
> Dirty heating and air conditioning equipment

If you notice these issues, it is important to evaluate potential sources of indoor pollution and take corrective action.[4]

Sources of Indoor Air Pollution

Many factors contribute to indoor air pollution, including:

Household Dust

Household dust consists of a mix of particles, including dead skin cells, fibers from carpets and furniture, pollen, and airborne pollutants. A significant portion of dust is composed of skin flakes, which shed continuously and accumulate in living spaces. Other sources include tracked-in soil, mold spores, and outdoor pollutants.

Dust Mites and Allergens

Dust mites thrive in warm, humid environments and feed on dead skin cells. They are one of the most common allergens and can trigger respiratory problems. Other common indoor allergens include pet dander and pollen, which can exacerbate allergy symptoms and asthma.

Ventilation and Airflow Issues

Poor ventilation can trap pollutants inside, leading to increased concentrations of allergens and airborne contaminants. Ensuring proper airflow by using ventilation systems, air purifiers, and regularly changing air filters can help improve indoor air quality.

Strategies to Improve Indoor Air Quality

To reduce dust, allergens, and airborne pollutants, consider the following strategies:

Cleaning and Maintenance

> **Use Microfiber Cloths:** These effectively trap dust and allergens instead of spreading them.
> **Vacuum with a HEPA Filter:** HEPA filters capture small particles that standard vacuums may recirculate into the air.
> **Wash Bedding Regularly:** Washing sheets, pillowcases, and blankets in hot water can kill dust mites and remove allergens.
> **Clean Air Ducts:** Dirty air ducts can harbor dust, mold, and bacteria. Professional cleaning can help maintain a healthier environment.

Controlling Humidity

>> **Use a Dehumidifier:** Keeping humidity levels between 40-50% can reduce mold growth and dust mite populations.

>> **Fix Leaks and Water Damage:** Moist areas encourage mold growth, which can release spores into the air.

Improving Ventilation

>> **Keep Windows Closed on High-Pollen Days:** While fresh air is beneficial, pollen and outdoor pollutants can enter through open windows.

>> **Change HVAC Filters Regularly:** Using high-efficiency filters in heating and cooling systems helps trap airborne particles and improve air circulation.

>> **Consider an Air Purifier:** Air purifiers with HEPA filters can help remove dust, pet dander, and other allergens from the air.

Who Is Most Affected by Poor Air Quality?

Certain individuals are more vulnerable to the effects of poor air quality, including:

>> Children and the elderly

>> Individuals with asthma, allergies, or respiratory conditions

>> People who spend a significant amount of time indoors

Taking proactive steps to improve air quality can benefit these individuals and create a healthier home environment.

Dust, allergens, and poor air quality can have a significant impact on health and well-being. By understanding the sources of indoor air pollution and implementing effective cleaning and maintenance strategies, you can create a cleaner, safer living environment. Regular cleaning, proper ventilation, and allergen control measures can help ensure that the air you breathe is as healthy as possible.

Harmful Chemicals That Contribute to Poor Air Quality

Common Household Chemicals and Their Effects

Many common household products and building materials contain harmful chemicals that contribute to indoor air pollution. These chemicals can off-gas into the air, leading to health problems ranging from mild irritation to serious respiratory issues.

Volatile Organic Compounds (VOCs)

VOCs are chemicals found in many household products, including paints, varnishes, cleaning supplies, and air fresheners. They can cause:

> Eye, nose, and throat irritation

> Headaches and dizziness

> Damage to the liver, kidneys, and central nervous system

Reducing VOC exposure involves using low-VOC or VOC-free products, ensuring proper ventilation, and avoiding aerosol sprays.[5]

Formaldehyde

Formaldehyde is a common indoor air pollutant found in pressed wood products, household cleaners, and even some textiles. It has been linked to respiratory issues and can trigger allergic reactions. To minimize exposure, choose formaldehyde-free furniture and avoid strong-smelling adhesives.[6]

Pesticides

Pesticides used in and around the home can linger in the air and on surfaces, posing risks to both humans and pets. Exposure to pesticides has been linked to:

>> Neurological damage
>> Endocrine system disruption
>> Respiratory problems[7]

Opt for natural pest control methods whenever possible and avoid excessive pesticide use indoors.

Cleaning Chemicals

Many household cleaning products contain harsh chemicals, including ammonia and chlorine. These can react with other airborne pollutants to form toxic compounds. Choosing natural cleaning alternatives, such as vinegar and baking soda, can help reduce indoor air pollution.[8]

Air Fresheners and Scented Candles

While they may make your home smell pleasant, air fresheners and scented candles often contain synthetic fragrances and VOCs that can contribute to indoor air pollution. These products release harmful chemicals that can irritate the respiratory system and worsen allergies or asthma.[9] Opt for natural alternatives such as essential oil diffusers or beeswax candles instead.

The Role of Off-Gassing in Poor Air Quality

Off-gassing occurs when chemicals in materials such as carpets, furniture, and paints release pollutants into the air. This process can be accelerated by heat and humidity. To minimize exposure, opt for natural materials and ensure proper ventilation in newly furnished or renovated spaces.[10]

Reducing exposure to harmful chemicals can significantly improve indoor air quality. By choosing safer household products, improving ventilation, and being mindful of off-gassing sources, you can create a healthier home environment for yourself and your family.

Additional Considerations

Allergens and Seasonal Allergies

Seasonal allergies are often triggered by airborne pollen, mold spores, and other allergens. Symptoms include sneezing, runny nose, and itchy eyes. To minimize seasonal allergies, consider:

> Keeping windows closed during peak pollen times

> Using high-efficiency particulate air (HEPA) filters

> Washing clothes and bedding frequently to remove allergens

> Showering after outdoor exposure to reduce pollen buildup

HVAC Systems and Air Quality

Your heating, ventilation, and air conditioning (HVAC) system plays a crucial role in maintaining indoor air quality. Best practices for HVAC maintenance include:

> Changing filters regularly

> Scheduling professional duct cleanings as needed

> Ensuring proper ventilation to prevent the buildup of indoor pollutants

Natural Air Freshener Alternatives

Instead of synthetic air fresheners that release harmful VOCs, consider natural alternatives such as:

> **Essential oil diffusers:** Provide a pleasant scent without harmful chemicals.

> **Beeswax candles:** Emit negative ions that help neutralize airborne pollutants.

> **Simmering citrus peels and herbs:** A natural way to add a fresh scent to your home.

The Role of Houseplants

Houseplants can help improve air quality by filtering toxins from the air.[11] Some of the best plants for air purification include:

> Snake plants

> Peace lilies

> Spider plants

The Importance of Proper Ventilation

Improving airflow helps remove indoor pollutants. Simple strategies include:

> Opening windows when outdoor air quality is good

> Using exhaust fans in kitchens and bathrooms

> Running an air purifier with a HEPA filter in high-traffic areas

Considering additional factors such as allergens, HVAC maintenance, and natural alternatives for air fresheners can further enhance indoor air quality. By making informed choices about household products and maintenance routines, you can create a healthier home environment for yourself and your family.

Did You Know? Fresher Air and Less Dust

Scented HVAC Filters: Adding a few drops of essential oil to your HVAC filter can circulate a pleasant aroma throughout your home. Scents like lavender, eucalyptus, or peppermint not only smell great but may also provide calming or energizing benefits.

Activated Charcoal — Nature's Air Filter: Activated charcoal works wonders for improving air quality. Through a process called adsorption (not absorption), its porous surface traps pollutants like VOCs, odors, and gases — leaving your indoor air cleaner and fresher.

Pollutant Powerhouse: Activated charcoal can help remove common household odors and pollutants such as:

> Cooking odors

> Pet smells

> Cigarette smoke

> Chemical fumes

> Volatile organic compounds (VOCs)

Dust-Defying Baseboards: For cleaner baseboards that resist dust buildup, wipe them down with a vinegar and water solution. Once dry, apply a thin layer of essential oil like lavender, eucalyptus, or cinnamon to help repel dust — and bugs!

Furniture Dust Spray Hack: Mix up this DIY dust-repelling solution for your furniture:

> ½ tsp olive oil (to repel dust)

> 1 tsp vinegar (to kill dust mites)

> ½ cup water

> 2 drops dish soap

> 10 drops lemon essential oil

Spray onto a microfiber cloth and wipe surfaces to keep dust at bay while leaving behind a fresh, clean scent.

Chapter Notes

1. U.S. Environmental Protection Agency. (2023, March 20). Biological pollutants' impact on indoor air quality. https://www.epa.gov/indoor-air-quality-iaq/biological-pollutants-impact-indoor-air-quality

2. Centers for Disease Control and Prevention. (2005, January 14). Case definitions for chemical poisoning. https://www.cdc.gov/mmwr/preview/mmwrhtml/rr5401a1.htm

3. U.S. Environmental Protection Agency. (2023, July 10). Indoor air quality. https://www.epa.gov/report-environment/indoor-air-quality

4. U.S. Environmental Protection Agency. (n.d.). The Inside Story: A Guide to Indoor Air Quality. Retrieved May 15, 2025, from https://www.epa.gov/indoor-air-quality-iaq/inside-story-guide-indoor-air-quality

5. U.S. Environmental Protection Agency. (n.d.). Volatile Organic Compounds' Impact on Indoor Air Quality. Retrieved May 15, 2025, from https://www.epa.gov/indoor-air-quality-iaq/volatile-organic-compounds-impact-indoor-air-quality

6. U.S. Environmental Protection Agency. (n.d.). Formaldehyde's Impact on Indoor Air Quality. Retrieved May 15, 2025, from https://www.epa.gov/indoor-air-quality-iaq/formaldehydes-impact-indoor-air-quality

7. U.S. Environmental Protection Agency. (n.d.). Pesticides' Impact on Indoor Air Quality. Retrieved May 15, 2025, from https://www.epa.gov/indoor-air-quality-iaq/pesticides-impact-indoor-air-quality

8. U.S. Environmental Protection Agency. (n.d.). Identifying Greener Cleaning Products. Retrieved May 15, 2025, from https://www.epa.gov/greenerproducts/identifying-greener-cleaning-products

9. U.S. Environmental Protection Agency. (n.d.). Volatile Organic Compounds' Impact on Indoor Air Quality. Retrieved May 15, 2025, from https://www.epa.gov/indoor-air-quality-iaq/volatile-organic-compounds-impact-indoor-air-quality

10. U.S. Environmental Protection Agency. (n.d.). Introduction to Indoor Air Quality. Retrieved May 15, 2025, from https://www.epa.gov/indoor-air-quality-iaq/introduction-indoor-air-quality

11. Wolverton, B. C., Johnson, A., & Bounds, K. (1989). Interior landscape plants for indoor air pollution abatement. National Aeronautics and Space Administration. Retrieved from https://ntrs.nasa.gov/api/citations/19930073077/downloads/19930073077.pdf

CHAPTER 9

Houseplants, Bugs & Outdoor Spaces

Houseplants and Indoor Air Quality

Houseplants do more than add beauty to our homes—they also improve air quality. In 1989, NASA, in collaboration with the Associated Landscape Contractors of America (ALCA), conducted a two-year study to determine how common household plants could purify indoor air. Led by Dr. B.C. Wolverton, Anne Johnson, and Keith Bounds, the study initially aimed to find solutions for purifying air on space stations. However, the findings had significant implications for improving air quality here on Earth.

The study revealed that houseplants can help remove volatile organic compounds (VOCs) from indoor air, including chemicals like formaldehyde, benzene, and trichloroethylene. These pollutants are found in everyday household materials such as paint, adhesives, building materials, and cleaning products. Since modern homes are often well-sealed with limited ventilation, these trapped pollutants can contribute to Sick Building Syndrome, leading to headaches, dizziness, and respiratory issues. Fortunately, certain plants excel at absorbing these toxins, making them a valuable addition to any home.[1]

Best Plants for Filtering Indoor Air

NASA's study identified several plants that are particularly effective at filtering specific chemicals:

For Formaldehyde Removal:

- » Bamboo Palm
- » Mother-in-Law's Tongue (Snake Plant)
- » Dracaena Warneckii
- » Peace Lily
- » Dracaena Marginata
- » Golden Pothos
- » Green Spider Plant

For Benzene Removal:

- » English Ivy
- » Gerbera Daisies
- » Pot Mums
- » Peace Lily
- » Bamboo Palm
- » Mother-in-Law's Tongue

For Trichloroethylene Removal:

- » Peace Lily
- » Gerbera Daisy
- » Bamboo Palm

General Indoor Air Purification Plants:

- » Heartleaf Philodendron *(Toxic to pets)*
- » Elephant Ear Philodendron *(Toxic to pets)*
- » Cornstalk Dracaena *(Toxic to pets)*

- ❯ English Ivy *(Toxic to pets)*
- ❯ Spider Plant *(Non-toxic to pets)*
- ❯ Janet Craig Dracaena *(Toxic to pets)*
- ❯ Weeping Fig *(Toxic to pets)*
- ❯ Golden Pothos *(Toxic to pets)*
- ❯ Peace Lily *(Toxic to pets)*
- ❯ Chinese Evergreen *(Toxic to pets)*
- ❯ Bamboo or Reed Palm *(Non-toxic to pets)*
- ❯ Red-Edged Dracaena *(Toxic to pets)*

While houseplants offer excellent air-purifying benefits, pet owners should be cautious about selecting varieties that are safe for their animals. Even non-toxic plants can cause vomiting or allergic reactions in pets, so monitoring interactions is essential.

Additional Benefits of Houseplants

Beyond air purification, houseplants provide several additional benefits, including:

1. Humidity Regulation

Plants naturally release moisture into the air through transpiration, helping to maintain a comfortable indoor humidity level. This is particularly useful in dry climates or during winter months when indoor heating reduces humidity.[1]

2. Stress Reduction and Well-Being

Studies suggest that the presence of greenery in indoor spaces can improve mood, reduce stress, and enhance overall well-being. The act of caring for plants has been linked to lower cortisol levels and increased feelings of relaxation.[2]

3. Improved Focus and Productivity

Indoor plants have been shown to boost concentration and cognitive function. This is why many offices incorporate greenery into their spaces—to enhance employee productivity and mental clarity.[3]

4. Natural Decor and Aesthetic Appeal

Houseplants serve as an inexpensive and sustainable way to enhance home decor. Their vibrant colors and unique shapes can add warmth and life to any indoor space.[4]

5. Connection to Nature

Having plants indoors provides a direct connection to nature, fostering a sense of tranquility and appreciation for the environment. This can be particularly valuable for individuals living in urban settings with limited access to outdoor green spaces.[5]

Choosing and Caring for Houseplants

Selecting the right houseplants depends on several factors, including available light, humidity levels, and maintenance preferences. Here are a few key tips for keeping houseplants healthy:

> » **Light Requirements:** Choose plants based on the natural light available in your home. Low-light plants, such as snake plants and pothos, thrive in shaded areas, while succulents and cacti need bright, direct sunlight.
> » **Watering Schedule:** Overwatering is one of the most common reasons plants die. It's important to research each plant's water needs and allow the soil to dry slightly between waterings.

> **Soil and Drainage:** Ensure that pots have drainage holes to prevent root rot. Using well-draining soil can also help maintain plant health.

> **Pest Prevention:** Keep an eye out for common houseplant pests such as spider mites, aphids, and fungus gnats. Natural remedies like neem oil or insecticidal soap can help control infestations.

> **Fertilization:** Some plants require occasional feeding with liquid or slow-release fertilizers to promote healthy growth.

Houseplants are much more than decorative elements; they play an important role in improving indoor air quality, regulating humidity, reducing stress, and enhancing well-being. By carefully selecting and maintaining the right plants, homeowners can create a healthier and more inviting indoor environment. Whether you choose air-purifying varieties, low-maintenance options, or simply plants that bring you joy, incorporating greenery into your living space offers a wide range of benefits for both physical and mental health.

A Natural Approach to Pest Control

Managing household pests without resorting to harsh chemicals is both environmentally friendly and safer for your family and pets. There are numerous natural solutions to prevent and eliminate common indoor and outdoor pests effectively. The key to success is consistency, cleanliness, and using natural deterrents tailored to specific pests.

Preventative Measures

One of the best ways to manage pests is to prevent them from becoming a problem in the first place. Here are some fundamental practices to keep your home and garden pest-free:

» **Keep Your Home Clean:** Pests are often attracted to food crumbs, standing water, and clutter. Regularly vacuum floors, wipe down counters, and avoid leaving dirty dishes in the sink. Wipe down baseboards with vinegar cleaning and go back over them with a cloth with either lavender oil or eucalyptus.

» **Seal Entry Points:** Inspect windows, doors, and any cracks in your home where pests might enter. Use caulk or weather stripping to seal gaps.

» **Remove Standing Water:** Mosquitoes breed in stagnant water. Regularly empty water from flower pots, birdbaths, and outdoor containers.

» **Proper Food Storage:** Store grains, pet food, and pantry items in airtight containers to prevent infestations.

Natural Indoor Pest Control Solutions

Ants

» **Lemon and Water Spray:** Mix equal parts lemon juice and water in a spray bottle and apply it to entry points and ant trails.

» **Vinegar:** Spraying white vinegar along baseboards and countertops disrupts their scent trails.

» **Cinnamon or Cayenne Pepper:** Sprinkling these spices near entry points repels ants naturally.

» **Boric Acid and Sugar Mix:** A mix of boric acid and sugar attracts and eliminates ants without harming humans or pets (use cautiously).

Silverfish

» **Remove Humidity:** Silverfish thrive in damp environments, so use dehumidifiers and keep areas dry.

> **Cedar and Bay Leaves:** Placing cedar shavings or bay leaves in cabinets and closets repels silverfish naturally.

> **Flour and Water Trap:** Mixing flour and water into a paste, then placing it on index cards, can help identify and reduce silverfish populations.

Fruit Flies

> **Apple Cider Vinegar Trap:** Fill a small bowl with apple cider vinegar and cover it with plastic wrap, poking small holes. Fruit flies enter but can't escape.

> **Basil and Cloves:** Keeping basil plants or a small dish of cloves in your kitchen naturally deters fruit flies.

> **Frequent Trash Removal:** Take out the garbage regularly and ensure fruit and vegetables are not overripe.

Mosquitoes

> **Essential Oils:** Cedar oil, rosemary oil, citronella, and eucalyptus oils can be applied to exposed skin or diffused indoors to repel mosquitoes.

> **Mosquito-Repelling Plants:** Grow citronella grass, rosemary, or marigolds near doors and patios.

> **Eliminate Standing Water:** Drain any sources of stagnant water to prevent breeding.

Spiders

> **Vinegar Spray:** A mix of equal parts vinegar and water can be sprayed in corners and around windows to deter spiders.

> **Keep Areas Clean:** Spiders thrive in cluttered spaces; frequent vacuuming and dusting will help keep them away.

>> **Citrus Peels:** Placing orange or lemon peels around the home naturally repels spiders.

Natural Outdoor Pest Control Solutions

Wasps

>> **Homemade Wasp Trap:** Cut the top third off a soda bottle, invert it, and tape it back onto the bottle's base. Fill it with fruit juice or soda to attract wasps.

>> **Peppermint Spray:** A mix of peppermint oil and water sprayed around eaves and entry points deters wasps from nesting.

>> **Remove Nests at Night:** If you must remove a nest, do so at night when wasps are less active. Carefully enclose the nest in a plastic bag and submerge it in water.

Flies

>> **Soak Tea Bags:** Place lemon ginger tea bags in a small dish and soak them in 91% rubbing alcohol for a few minutes to release their natural fly-repelling scent.

>> **Place Around the Porch:** Set the soaked tea bags in fly-prone areas like tables, railings, or corners. Use small containers if needed to keep them from blowing away.

>> **Refresh as Needed:** Re-soak or replace tea bags once they dry out or lose scent. The combo of citrus, ginger, and alcohol helps mask odors that attract flies.

Slugs

>> **Beer Traps:** Place shallow bowls filled with stale beer in gardens; slugs are attracted to the yeast and will drown.

> **Copper Tape:** Creating a barrier of copper tape around plants prevents slugs from reaching them.
> **Eggshells or Diatomaceous Earth:** Sprinkling crushed eggshells or diatomaceous earth (DE), around plants acts as a deterrent. Diatomaceous earth is a naturally occurring, soft, siliceous sedimentary rock that crumbles into a fine, powdery substance. Food-grade DE is widely available for purchase both online and in physical stores.

Ladybugs

> **Seal Entry Points:** Ladybugs enter homes through small cracks. Sealing gaps around windows and doors prevents infestations.
> **Use a Shop Vacuum:** If ladybugs enter your home, gently vacuum them up and release them outside.
> **Install a Ladybug House:** Provide an alternative shelter outdoors to attract them away from your home. They are available at garden centers, home improvement stores, and online retailers like Amazon. Place the house in a sunny, sheltered spot near your garden, away from strong winds. Position it near plants that attract ladybugs, such as marigolds, dill, or yarrow. Adding some dried leaves or small twigs inside can make the house more inviting. By giving ladybugs a cozy home outdoors, you can naturally deter them from moving indoors.

Asian Ladybugs (Ladybirds)

> **Set the Trap:** Fill a zip-lock bag with 1 cup of cornstarch, shake to coat the inside, and tape it to a window where ladybugs tend to gather—leaving a small opening at the top.

> **Capture Naturally:** The cornstarch attracts and traps the ladybugs without harming them. Once inside, the powder restricts their movement, making it hard for them to escape.

> **Dispose and Prevent:** When enough have gathered, seal and dispose of the bag far from your home. Check the trap regularly and seal window or door cracks to prevent future invasions.

Managing pests naturally requires a proactive approach, but it is entirely possible without relying on harmful chemicals. By combining cleanliness, physical barriers, and natural deterrents, you can keep your indoor and outdoor spaces pest-free while maintaining a safe and eco-friendly environment for your family and pets.

Creating a Holistic and Sustainable Home Environment

In addition to maintaining air-purifying houseplants and using natural pest control methods, there are other important considerations to ensure a healthier, more sustainable home. These aspects encompass water conservation, non-toxic cleaning, eco-friendly furnishings, and overall indoor wellness.

Water Conservation for Indoor and Outdoor Plants

Sustainable water use is crucial for maintaining houseplants and outdoor gardens. Here are some simple yet effective water conservation tips:

> **Use Collected Rainwater:** Set up a rain barrel to collect rainwater for watering plants. This reduces reliance on tap water and is free of chlorine and other chemicals.

> **Water During Optimal Times:** Watering in the early morning or late evening prevents rapid evaporation and allows better absorption.

> » **Choose Drought-Tolerant Plants:** If water conservation is a priority, consider indoor plants like succulents, snake plants, and zamioculcas zamiifolia plants that require less frequent watering.
> » **Mulch Outdoor Gardens:** Using mulch around plants retains moisture, suppresses weeds, and reduces the need for frequent watering.

Non-Toxic Cleaning Alternatives

Many conventional cleaning products contain harsh chemicals that contribute to indoor air pollution. By switching to natural cleaning solutions, you can improve air quality and reduce exposure to toxins.

DIY Non-Toxic Cleaning Solutions:

> » **All-Purpose Cleaner:** Mix equal parts white vinegar and water with a few drops of essential oil (such as lemon or tea tree oil) for a fresh scent.
> » **Glass Cleaner:** Use a mixture of white vinegar and water for streak-free windows and mirrors.
> » **Baking Soda Scrub:** Combine baking soda with water to create a paste for scrubbing sinks, bathtubs, and countertops.
> » **Lemon and Salt for Cutting Boards:** Sprinkle salt on cutting boards and rub with a lemon to naturally disinfect and deodorize.

Eco-Friendly Furnishings and Materials

Selecting sustainable and non-toxic materials for your home can reduce your environmental footprint while improving indoor health.

> » **Opt for Low-VOC Paints and Finishes:** Volatile organic compounds (VOCs) in traditional paints and finishes can emit harmful fumes. Choose low-VOC or VOC-free alternatives.

> **Choose Sustainable Fabrics:** Opt for organic cotton, bamboo, or linen for curtains, upholstery, and bedding to avoid synthetic chemical treatments.

> **Select FSC-Certified Wood:** The Forest Stewardship Council (FSC) certification ensures that wood products are sourced from responsibly managed forests.

> **Repurpose and Upcycle:** Instead of purchasing new furniture, consider refinishing, repainting, or repurposing old furniture to reduce waste.

Improving Indoor Air Quality Beyond Plants

Houseplants play a crucial role in improving air quality, but additional strategies can further enhance indoor wellness.

> **Use Air Purifiers:** High-efficiency particulate air (HEPA) filters can remove allergens, dust, and pollutants from the air.

> **Increase Ventilation:** Open windows regularly to allow fresh air to circulate and prevent indoor pollutants from accumulating.

> **Avoid Synthetic Fragrances:** Air fresheners and scented candles often contain artificial chemicals. Opt for essential oil diffusers or naturally scented soy or beeswax candles instead.

> **Maintain Proper Humidity Levels:** Using a humidifier or dehumidifier as needed can prevent mold growth and create a more comfortable indoor climate.

Sustainable Waste Management

Reducing household waste helps minimize environmental impact and supports sustainability efforts.

> **Compost Organic Waste:** Kitchen scraps, coffee grounds, and plant trimmings can be composted to enrich garden soil.

> **Recycle Responsibly:** Follow local recycling guidelines to ensure that plastic, glass, paper, and metal are properly processed.

> **Reduce Single-Use Plastics:** Replace disposable plastic items with reusable alternatives, such as stainless steel straws, cloth shopping bags, and glass containers.

> **Donate or Repurpose Unwanted Items:** Before discarding furniture, clothes, or household goods, consider donating them to local charities or upcycling them for new uses.

By incorporating these additional considerations into your home care routine, you can create a healthier, more sustainable living environment. From conserving water and choosing non-toxic cleaning solutions to selecting eco-friendly furnishings and improving indoor air quality, small changes can lead to significant benefits for both your household and the planet. A holistic approach to home maintenance ensures that your space remains safe, comfortable, and environmentally responsible.

Did You Know? Fun Facts for Happier House-plants, Outdoor Spaces, and Bug-Free Living

Ant Control Trick: To keep ants away (indoors or out), mix 1 cup of powdered sugar with ¼ cup of baking soda. Sprinkle the mixture along baseboards or near outdoor ant nests. The sugar attracts them, and the baking soda disrupts their digestive system.

Mosquito, Tick, and Flea Defense: Sprinkle a mixture of 10 teaspoons of ground coffee (not decaf!) and 1 teaspoon of cayenne pepper around your yard to deter these pesky insects.

Hydrogen Peroxide for Fleas and Gnats: A light spray of 3% hydrogen peroxide in your yard can help keep fleas, ticks, and gnats at bay. It's a simple, pet-safe solution for outdoor areas.

Outdoor Fly Repellent: Soak lemon ginger tea bags in 91% rubbing alcohol for 2-3 minutes, then hang the bags around your porch or patio to help ward off flies.

Spider Solution: For a pet-friendly spider deterrent, use peppermint extract (not peppermint oil, which can be unsafe for pets). Soak a cotton swab in peppermint extract and place it wherever spiders like to hide.

Chapter Notes

1. Wolverton, B. C., Johnson, A., & Bounds, K. (1989). Interior landscape plants for indoor air pollution abatement. National Aeronautics and Space Administration (NASA), Stennis Space Center. https://ntrs.nasa.gov/api/citations/19930073077/downloads/19930073077.pdf

2. Lee, M. S., Lee, J., Park, B. J., & Miyazaki, Y. (2015). Interaction with indoor plants may reduce psychological and physiological stress by suppressing autonomic nervous system activity in young adults: A randomized crossover study. Journal of Physiological Anthropology, 34(1), 21. https://doi.org/10.1186/s40101-015-0060-8

3. Nieuwenhuis, M., Knight, C., Postmes, T., & Haslam, S. A. (2014). The relative benefits of green versus lean office space: Three field experiments. Journal of Experimental Psychology: Applied, 20(3), 199–214. https://doi.org/10.1037/xap0000024

4. Bringslimark, T., Hartig, T., & Patil, G. G. (2009). The psychological benefits of indoor plants: A critical review of the experimental literature. Journal of Environmental Psychology, 29(4), 422–433. https://doi.org/10.1016/j.jenvp.2009.05.001

5. Kaplan, R., & Kaplan, S. (1989). The experience of nature: A psychological perspective. Cambridge University Press.

PART 3
Labels, Ingredients & Sustainability

CHAPTER 10

Decoding Labels & Avoiding Toxic Ingredients

What's Really in Your Cleaning Products?

Health problems have been linked to environmental toxins in the home, affecting everything from respiratory issues to pediatric cancer. These toxins enter our bodies through skin absorption and inhalation. In fact, the EPA consistently ranks indoor air quality among the top five environmental risks to human health.[1]

Unlike food, beverages, or drugs, cleaning products are not regulated by the U.S. Food and Drug Administration. While the U.S. Environmental Protection Agency (EPA) requires manufacturers to list active disinfectants or harmful ingredients, companies are only obligated to disclose "chemicals of known concern." Shockingly, most chemicals used in everyday cleaning products have never been tested for safety, nor are manufacturers required to test them.[2]

As a parent, I have spent years searching for truly non-toxic cleaning products. I've tested green brands, aiming to find options that are effective, pleasant-smelling, and, most importantly, safe for my family. However, separating genuinely non-toxic products from those simply marketed as "green" can be tricky. The term "green" is often just a marketing tactic rather than a verified safety standard.

The Federal Trade Commission (FTC) is currently reviewing and updating its *Green Guides*, which aim to prevent misleading environmental marketing claims. Until those updates take effect, consumers need to be informed.

According to the FTC's Consumer Resource for Sorting Out Green Claims:

> "Claims that a product is 'environmentally friendly,' 'safe,' or 'eco-friendly' are vague and often misleading. All products have some environmental impact, and these phrases do not provide the specific details needed to compare products."[3]

Finding Safer Cleaning Products

If you want truly safer products, understanding ingredient labels is crucial—especially when terms like "plant-based materials" are used without further clarification. The National Institutes of Health (NIH) maintains a database of chemicals and their health effects, which can be a helpful resource.

A good rule of thumb: If you can't pronounce an ingredient, it's worth researching before bringing it into your home.

Decoding Labels: What to Watch For

Many cleaning product labels use misleading terms or fail to disclose harmful ingredients. Here's a guide to understanding what's really in your cleaning supplies.

Problematic Ingredients & Terms

> » **Active Ingredient:** Typically an antimicrobial pesticide added to kill bacteria, viruses, or mold. These are often unnecessary and hazardous.
> » **Antibacterial:** Indicates the presence of pesticides. Overuse can contribute to antibiotic resistance.
> » **Biodegradable:** Unregulated term. Some ingredients break down safely, but others degrade into harmful substances.
> » **Chlorine-Free/Bleach Alternative:** May contain oxygen bleach instead, which is still a respiratory irritant.

> **Combustible/Flammable:** Can pose a fire hazard; store away from heat sources.

> **Corrosive/Caustic:** Can cause chemical burns (e.g., oven cleaners, drain openers, bleach).

> **Do Not Induce Vomiting:** Indicates ingestion could cause severe harm or death. Call Poison Control immediately if ingested (1-800-222-1222).

> **Essential Oils:** Natural but not always safe. Some cause skin irritation or allergic reactions.

> **Fragrance:** A single word that can represent dozens of undisclosed chemicals. Avoid if possible.

> **Irritant:** Can cause skin, eye, or lung inflammation.

> **Natural/Plant-Based:** Unregulated and often meaningless. May still contain harmful chemicals.

> **Non-Toxic:** Unregulated term that does not guarantee safety.

> **Optical Brightener:** Found in laundry detergents; coats fabrics and can irritate skin.

> **Organic:** Unregulated in cleaning products. Only the USDA Certified Organic label ensures compliance.

> **Pesticide:** Used in antibacterial cleaners; harmful to people and pets.

> **Phosphate-Free:** Now standard in detergents due to environmental bans, making this label mostly meaningless.

> **Solvent:** Can be toxic; many release harmful volatile organic compounds (VOCs).

> **Surfactant:** Necessary for cleaning but varies in safety. Some are highly toxic to aquatic life.

> **Volatile Organic Compounds (VOCs):** Air pollutants linked to respiratory issues and smog formation.

Understanding Greenwashing

Many brands exploit consumer concerns by marketing their products as "green" when they are not. This deceptive practice is called greenwashing. Greenwashing is a deceptive marketing practice where a company exaggerates or falsely claims its products, services, or overall operations are environmentally friendly to appeal to eco-conscious consumers. Instead of making genuine sustainability efforts, greenwashing focuses more on appearing eco-friendly rather than being eco-friendly.[4]

How to spot greenwashing:

>> A product claims to be "non-toxic" on the front but has hazard warnings on the back.
>> A label lists one organic ingredient but contains several synthetic chemicals.
>> A product promotes vague claims like "eco-friendly" without specifying why.

To avoid falling for greenwashing, look for products that list all ingredients and provide detailed explanations of their claims.

Decoding Symbols on Cleaning Products

Symbol	What It Means
☠ **Extreme Hazard**	Found on antifreeze, paint removers, and insecticides. Avoid these in the home.
⚠ **Highly Toxic**	Found in oven cleaners, drain cleaners, and bleach. Can cause severe burns.

⚠ **Medium Hazard**	Found in flea sprays, toilet cleaners, and polishes containing neurotoxic chemicals.
⚠ **Low to Medium Hazard**	Found in glass cleaners, all-purpose cleaners, and some detergents.

Green Label Primer: Trusted Certifications

Certification	What It Means
USDA Organic	Indicates 95% organic ingredients; certified free of synthetic pesticides and fertilizers.
Leaping Bunny	No animal testing conducted on the product or its ingredients.
Green Seal	Environmentally sound cleaning products from manufacturing to disposal.
Forest Stewardship Council (FSC)	Certifies sustainably sourced wood and paper.
Recyclable ♻	Indicates use of easily recyclable materials.
Post-Consumer Waste Recycled	Made from recycled materials, reducing landfill waste.

Smart Shopping: Reducing Waste & Exposure

> **Buy in Bulk:** Reduce plastic waste by refilling smaller bottles.
> **Skip Fragrances:** Choose unscented or naturally scented products.
> **Use Simple Ingredients:** Vinegar, baking soda, and lemon work just as well as many commercial cleaners.

The Bottom Line

Understanding product labels is key to protecting your home and health. Marketing claims can be misleading, so always read ingredient lists carefully. Stick to brands that are transparent about their ingredients and opt for products certified by reputable third-party organizations.

Your choices matter—not just for your family's health, but for the environment as well.

Chapter Notes

1. U.S. Environmental Protection Agency. (n.d.). Indoor Air Quality Backgrounder: The Basics [PDF]. Retrieved from https://www.epa.gov/sites/default/files/2015-09/documents/backgrounder.pdf
2. U.S. Environmental Protection Agency. (n.d.). Introduction to Indoor Air Quality. Retrieved from https://www.epa.gov/indoor-air-quality-iaq/introduction-indoor-air-quality
3. Federal Trade Commission. (n.d.). Green Guides. Retrieved from https://www.ftc.gov/news-events/topics/truth-advertising/green-guides
4. FSC. (2024, October 17). What is greenwashing? Exposing deceptive tactics. Retrieved May 15, 2025, from https://fsc.org/en/blog/what-is-greenwashing

CHAPTER 11

General Cleaning Recipes

Maintaining a clean home doesn't have to mean using harsh chemicals. Many natural ingredients, such as castile soap, witch hazel, hydrogen peroxide, and even shaving cream, can be used to create effective, eco-friendly cleaning solutions. Below are a variety of cleaning recipes that use these ingredients to keep your home spotless.

All-Purpose Cleaners

Castile Soap All-Purpose Cleaner

A mild yet effective solution for removing dirt, grime, and stains on various surfaces.

Ingredients:

> ¼ cup liquid castile soap
> 1 ¾ cups water
> 1 tablespoon white vinegar
> 10-15 drops essential oil (optional; lemon or tea tree oil work well)

Instructions:

1. Mix all ingredients in a spray bottle and shake to combine.
2. Spray onto surfaces such as countertops, tables, and bathroom sinks.
3. Wipe clean with a microfiber cloth or sponge.

Tip: For extra cleaning power, add a teaspoon of baking soda to tackle tougher spots.

Witch Hazel All-Purpose Cleaner

Witch hazel is a natural astringent with mild antiseptic properties.

Ingredients:

- ½ cup witch hazel
- ½ cup water
- 1 tablespoon white vinegar (optional, for extra cleaning power)
- 10-15 drops essential oil (like lemon, lavender, or tea tree oil)

Instructions:

1. Mix all ingredients in a spray bottle.
2. Shake well before each use.
3. Spray on countertops, tables, and other surfaces and wipe with a clean cloth.

Glass & Mirror Cleaners

Streak-Free Glass Cleaner

Hydrogen peroxide and rubbing alcohol help dissolve grime without streaking.

Ingredients:

- ¼ cup hydrogen peroxide
- ¼ cup water
- 1 tablespoon white vinegar
- 1 tablespoon cornstarch (optional, for extra cleaning power)

Instructions:

1. Mix all ingredients in a spray bottle.
2. Shake well before using.
3. Spray on glass surfaces and wipe with a microfiber cloth or newspaper.

Bathroom Cleaners

Castile Soap Bathroom Cleaner

Great for tubs, sinks, and toilets.

Ingredients:

- ¼ cup castile soap
- ¼ cup white vinegar
- 1 ½ cups water
- 10 drops tea tree essential oil (optional, for antimicrobial properties)

Instructions:

1. Mix ingredients in a spray bottle and shake well.
2. Spray on sinks, tubs, and toilet bowls.
3. Let sit for 5-10 minutes, then scrub and rinse thoroughly.

Tip: For toilet stains, pour directly into the bowl and scrub with a toilet brush.

Disinfecting Bathroom Spray (Rubbing Alcohol Based)

Disinfects and cuts through soap scum and mildew.

Ingredients:

- ½ cup rubbing alcohol (70% or 90%)
- ½ cup water
- 1 tablespoon white vinegar
- 5-10 drops tea tree or lavender essential oil

Instructions:

1. Mix ingredients in a spray bottle.
2. Spray on bathroom surfaces and wipe clean.

Kitchen Cleaners

Dish Soap

A natural, chemical-free alternative for washing dishes.

Ingredients:

- ½ cup liquid castile soap
- ¼ cup water
- 1 tablespoon white vinegar
- 1 teaspoon essential oil (optional; lemon, lavender, or peppermint work well)

Instructions:

1. Combine ingredients in a small bottle or jar and shake to mix.
2. Use a small amount for washing dishes.

Tip: Add a few drops directly to the dishwasher's soap compartment.

Cutting Board Sanitizer (Hydrogen Peroxide Based)

Kills bacteria left behind from raw meat and vegetables.

Ingredients:

- ¼ cup hydrogen peroxide
- Water

Instructions:

1. Pour hydrogen peroxide onto the cutting board.
2. Let it bubble for a few minutes.
3. Scrub and rinse with warm water.

Carpet & Upholstery Cleaner

Carpet & Upholstery Stain Remover

A gentle and effective cleaner for pet-friendly homes.

Ingredients:

- ¼ cup liquid castile soap
- 1 cup water
- 1 tablespoon white vinegar
- 10-15 drops essential oil (optional; lavender or eucalyptus work well)

Instructions:

1. Mix ingredients in a spray bottle.
2. Spray onto stains and let sit for 5-10 minutes.
3. Blot with a clean cloth or sponge.
4. Rinse with water and blot again until the stain is gone.

Shaving Cream Carpet Cleaner

Shaving cream is surprisingly effective at lifting stains.

Ingredients:

- ¼ cup shaving cream (non-gel)
- 1 tablespoon white vinegar
- ½ cup warm water

Instructions:

1. Mix the shaving cream, vinegar, and water.
2. Apply directly to stains.
3. Blot and rinse with water.

Laundry & Fabric Care We should mention borax and washing soda

Laundry Detergent

A safe, eco-friendly detergent for sensitive skin.

Ingredients:

- ¼ cup liquid castile soap
- ¼ cup baking soda (optional, for stain-fighting power)
- 1 tablespoon white vinegar (optional, for fabric softening)

Instructions:

1. Add castile soap directly to the washing machine.
2. If using baking soda, add it to the drum.
3. Run your wash as usual.

Specialty Cleaners

Pet Shampoo

A gentle, natural shampoo for pets with sensitive skin.

Ingredients:

- ¼ cup liquid castile soap
- 1 cup warm water
- 1 tablespoon coconut oil (optional, for moisturizing)
- 10 drops lavender or chamomile essential oil (optional, for calming effects)

Instructions:

1. Mix ingredients in a bottle.

2. Wet your pet's fur and apply the shampoo.

3. Massage into their coat and rinse thoroughly.

Stainless Steel Cleaner (Epsom Salt Based)

Removes streaks and shines stainless steel appliances.

Ingredients:

> ¼ cup Epsom salt
> ¼ cup olive oil or vegetable oil

Instructions:

1. Mix ingredients into a paste.

2. Rub onto the stainless steel surface.

3. Buff with a clean cloth.

BONUS: A Cleaner Home with DIY Slime

DIY Cleaning Slime: Did you know you can make your own slime that's perfect for cleaning hard-to-reach areas? With just a few simple ingredients, you can create a fun, effective tool for tackling dust and crumbs.

What You'll Need:

> 4 oz Elmer's white glue
> ¼ cup water
> 1 tsp baking soda
> 2 tbsp contact lens solution (or ½ tsp borax in ½ cup hot water)
> Optional: A few drops of food coloring for a fun touch

How to Make It:

1. Mix the glue and water in a bowl.

2. Add food coloring if desired and stir well.

3. Stir in the baking soda, then slowly add the contact lens solution (or borax solution).

4. Stir until the mixture thickens, then knead it with your hands until you have a slime-like consistency.

How to Use Your Cleaning Slime:

> **Dust & Crumb Removal:** Perfect for cleaning keyboards, car consoles, and between furniture.

> **Crevice Cleaning:** Its flexible texture makes it great for squeezing into tight spots and pulling out dirt.

> **Surface Cleaning:** Ideal for sticky or dusty surfaces — it grabs residue without leaving anything behind.

Bonus Tip: Store your slime in an airtight container to keep it fresh for repeated use!

———

These fun and natural cleaning recipes will help you maintain a fresh, chemical-free home while being kind to the environment. Enjoy your clean, green home!

CHAPTER 12

Sustainability Beyond Cleaning

A truly eco-friendly home goes beyond just using natural cleaning solutions—it involves making conscious choices that reduce waste, conserve resources, and support a sustainable lifestyle. In this final chapter, we'll explore how to minimize plastic waste, embrace sustainable storage options, and develop long-term habits for a greener home.

Reducing Plastic Waste in Household Products

Plastic waste is a major environmental issue, with single-use plastics contributing significantly to pollution. By reducing plastic use in household products, we can minimize our environmental impact while creating a healthier home. Here are some strategies to cut down on plastic waste:

> **Choose Plastic-Free Packaging:** Look for household and cleaning products packaged in glass, metal, or compostable materials instead of plastic. Brands that use biodegradable or reusable containers are ideal.

> **Buy in Bulk:** Purchasing cleaning ingredients like baking soda, vinegar, and castile soap in bulk reduces the need for single-use plastic packaging.

> **Switch to Bar and Powdered Products:** Many cleaning and personal care products, such as dish soap, laundry detergent, and shampoos, are available in bar or powdered form, reducing plastic bottle waste.

> » **Opt for Refillable Cleaning Products:** Many companies now offer refill stations or subscription services that provide refills in sustainable packaging.
> » **Ditch Disposable Cleaning Wipes:** Instead of single-use disinfectant wipes, use reusable cloths with a DIY disinfecting spray.

Sustainable Storage and Refillable Options

Storage solutions play a key role in maintaining a sustainable home. Choosing eco-friendly materials and refillable options helps minimize waste while keeping your space organized and efficient.

> » **Glass and Stainless-Steel Containers:** Store homemade cleaning solutions in glass spray bottles or stainless-steel dispensers instead of plastic ones.
> » **Mason Jars and Reused Jars:** Repurpose old glass jars for storage of powders, detergents, and DIY cleaners.
> » **Silicone and Fabric Storage Bags:** Replace plastic storage bags with reusable silicone or fabric alternatives for storing sponges, brushes, and small household items.
> » **DIY Cleaning Pods and Concentrates:** Create concentrated cleaning solutions that can be diluted in water as needed, reducing packaging waste and storage space.
> » **Refill Stations and Bulk Stores:** Visit refill stations or zero-waste shops for dish soap, laundry detergent, and multi-purpose cleaners in bulk.

Long-Term Habits for a Greener Home

Sustainability isn't just about one-time changes—it's about cultivating long-term habits that support an eco-conscious lifestyle. Here are some practices to integrate into your daily routine:

> **Reduce, Reuse, Recycle:** Follow the three R's by minimizing consumption, repurposing items whenever possible, and recycling properly.

> **Compost Organic Waste:** Set up a compost bin for food scraps and biodegradable materials to reduce landfill waste.

> **Use Energy-Efficient Cleaning Methods:** Wash clothes in cold water, air dry laundry, and clean with microfiber cloths to conserve energy.

> **Support Sustainable Brands:** Choose companies that prioritize sustainability, ethical sourcing, and minimal waste packaging.

> **Adopt Minimalist Living:** Reduce excess clutter and consumption by investing in high-quality, long-lasting products rather than disposable or trendy items.

> **Educate and Inspire Others:** Share your sustainable habits with friends and family, and encourage them to make eco-friendly choices.

Living sustainably extends beyond just cleaning—it's about making conscious choices every day that contribute to a healthier home and a healthier planet. By reducing plastic waste, choosing refillable and sustainable storage options, and developing long-term eco-friendly habits, we can create a lifestyle that benefits both ourselves and future generations. Small changes, when made consistently, can have a significant impact. Let's commit to sustainability beyond cleaning and build a greener future together.

A Cleaner Home, A Healthier Planet

As we reach the end of this journey, I hope you feel empowered with the knowledge and tools to transform the way you clean your home. Choosing eco-friendly cleaning methods isn't just about replacing harsh chemicals with natural alternatives; it's about redefining what it means to have a truly clean home—one that is safe for you, your family, and the environment.

Small Steps, Big Impact

Throughout this book, we've explored why conventional cleaning products pose a threat to our health and our planet. We've uncovered the simple yet powerful ingredients that can replace toxic cleaners, and we've walked through every room in the house, learning how to tackle dirt, grime, and bacteria without harming ourselves or the environment. We've also taken a deeper dive into how to identify greenwashing and make informed choices that extend beyond just cleaning.

If there's one thing I hope you take away, it's that small, mindful changes add up. Every time you swap a chemical-laden cleaner for a natural one, choose a reusable cloth over disposable wipes, or support a sustainable brand, you are making a difference. Every action—no matter how small—contributes to a larger movement toward a healthier home and a more sustainable world.

The Future of Cleaning Is in Our Hands

Eco-friendly cleaning isn't just a trend; it's a necessity. The choices we make today will shape the future for generations to come. As more people become aware of the impact of conventional cleaning products, demand for safer alternatives will continue to grow. By leading the way in your own home, you set an example for others, showing that safe and effective cleaning doesn't require sacrificing convenience or results.

This journey doesn't end with the last page of this book. As new research, innovations, and sustainable solutions emerge, there will always be opportunities to refine and improve the way we care for our homes. I encourage you to stay curious, keep learning, and share your knowledge with others. The more we spread awareness and support eco-friendly practices, the greater our collective impact will be.

A Personal Commitment

Writing this book has been a deeply personal endeavor for me. My experience in the cleaning industry opened my eyes to the dangers of conventional products, and my mission has been to help others make safer choices without feeling overwhelmed. I am grateful that you've taken the time to explore these ideas with me, and I hope this book has provided you with the confidence to embrace a more sustainable way of cleaning.

If you ever find yourself unsure or needing a refresher, come back to these pages. Revisit the recipes, remind yourself of the why behind these changes, and know that each step you take matters. Whether you implement one change or completely overhaul your cleaning routine, you are making a positive difference.

Moving Forward

So, what's next? Start where you can. Try a DIY all-purpose cleaner, swap out synthetic air fresheners for natural alternatives, or commit to using fewer disposable cleaning products. Share your journey with friends and family—change is contagious, and your choices might inspire others to make the switch, too.

As Margaret Mead so wisely said, *"Never doubt that a small group of thoughtful, committed citizens can change the world; indeed, it is the only thing that ever has."*

Thank you for joining me on this path toward a cleaner, healthier, and more sustainable home. Let's continue making choices that protect not only our families but also the planet we call home.

PRODUCT PURCHASING GUIDE

This guide outlines the preferred ingredients and products for natural, green cleaning. The following items are recommended based on purity, performance, and accessibility. None of the brands listed are affiliated with multi-level marketing companies.

Essential Oils

What to Look For:

> **Purity:** Avoid oils with added chemicals, synthetic ingredients, or fillers. Pure oils typically list the botanical name (e.g., *Lavandula officinalis* for lavender).

> **Aroma:** Quality oils should smell strong and natural, without artificial, unpleasant, or alcohol-like notes.

> **Brand Reputation:** Choose companies that offer transparency, quality guarantees, and third-party testing such as GC-MS (Gas Chromatography-Mass Spectrometry).

> **Label Information:** Look for botanical name, country of origin, and a clear purity statement.

> **Other Considerations:** Pay attention to how plants are grown (wildcrafted or organic). Be cautious of oils priced significantly below competitors—they may be diluted or lower quality.

Recommended Brands:

> Plant Therapy
> Thrive
> Eden Garden
> Rocky Mountain Oils

> Far & Wild
> Floracopeia
> Simply Earth

Witch Hazel

What to Look For:

> Choose **alcohol-free** versions.
> Check ingredient lists for absence of harsh chemicals, parabens, phthalates, and gluten.

Recommended Brands:

> Dickinson
> Thayers

Castile Soap

What to Look For:

> **Ingredients:** True castile soap is made from 100% plant-based oils like olive, coconut, or hemp—not animal fats.
> **Certifications:** Look for USDA Organic, Fair Trade, or Cruelty-Free.
> **Skin & Scent Needs:** Choose according to skin sensitivity and scent preferences (natural or unscented options available).

Recommended Brands:

> Dr. Bronner
> Kirks
> California Baby
> Carolina Castile Soap

> The Honest Company
> Ecover

Specialty Soaps and Powders

Fels-Naptha: An American brand of laundry soap originally created in 1893. It was historically used to treat poison ivy due to its active ingredient naphtha. Today, it is still effective for laundry pre-treatment and stain removal.

Bon Ami: A gentle scouring powder. The name means "Good Friend" in French. It's suitable for non-toxic cleaning of sinks, cookware, and tubs.

Borax (Sodium Borate)

While borax is naturally occurring, it is still a chemical compound ($Na_2B_4O_7$). It's often marketed as green but should be handled with care.

Note: "Natural" does not always mean "non-toxic" or "harmless." (Source: David Suzuki Foundation, Healthline)

Laundry Soap

Most conventional laundry soaps contain surfactants, optical brighteners, artificial fragrances, and dyes. Look instead for plant-based or mineral-based alternatives that are free of these harsh additives.

Rubbing Alcohol

> **70% Isopropyl Alcohol:** Best for general cleaning and disinfecting. The water content helps alcohol penetrate cell walls more effectively.
> **90%+ Isopropyl Alcohol:** Ideal for cleaning electronics and removing sticky residue, thanks to quick evaporation.

Hydrogen Peroxide

An effective disinfectant and bleach alternative.

> » Common household use: 3% solution
> » Higher concentrations are available but should be used with care and for specific applications only. (See: Nordchem guide on hydrogen peroxide percentages: nordchem.co.uk/blogs/hydrogen-peroxide-1/differences-hydrogen-peroxide-solution)

Epsom Salt

Useful for tile and grout cleaning, drain unclogging, and odor removal.

Recommended Brands:

> » SaltWorks Ultra Epsom (medium grain)
> » Dr Teal's
> » Sky Organics

Uses:

> » Mix with castile soap to scrub surfaces.
> » Pour into drains to help dissolve grease and hair buildup.

Citric Acid Powder

A highly versatile and natural cleaner used to remove:

> » Mineral deposits
> » Limescale
> » Rust
> » Hard water stains
> » Appliance buildup (coffee makers, dishwashers)

Grades of Citric Acid:

> **Laboratory Grade:** Scientific and industrial use
> **Food Grade:** Best for household use (cleaning and culinary)
> **Pharmaceutical Grade:** Used in medications

Baking Soda & Baking Powder

Common household staples used in natural cleaning.

> **Baking soda** is especially helpful as a gentle abrasive and deodorizer.
> **Baking powder** is less common in cleaning use but can serve as a mild leavening or scrubbing agent.

ABOUT THE AUTHOR

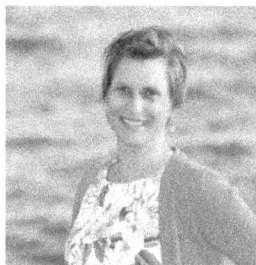

Cathy Mails is a pioneer in natural, eco-friendly home cleaning and the owner of Sea Green Natural Cleaning. With over 50 years of experience in the cleaning industry, Cathy has developed a deep, specialized knowledge of natural cleaning solutions that create healthier, toxin-free living environments.

Her commitment to excellence and sustainability has earned Sea Green multiple accolades, including Topsail's Top Choice People's Choice Award and 1st Place Favorite Cleaning Organization. Sea Green Natural is also the only ocean-friendly certified green business in North Carolina. Having been in the hospitality and cleaning industry for over 50 years, Cathy's passion extends beyond just cleaning—she is on a mission to educate homeowners about the benefits of natural, non-toxic cleaning practices that promote well-being and environmental responsibility.

As an author, Cathy shares her wealth of expertise, offering readers practical strategies for maintaining a cleaner, healthier home without relying on harmful chemicals. Whether through her company or her writing, she continues to lead the way in redefining what it means to truly clean green.

ABOUT SMART PUBLISHING

Ready to turn your book dream into reality?

Whether you're an aspiring author or a seasoned entrepreneur, Smart Publishing is here to guide you to success. With our proven expertise and 100% success rate in creating bestselling authors, your book will receive the recognition it deserves.

Don't let uncertainty hold you back. Take the first step toward becoming a bestselling author and dominating your marketplace. Scan the QR code to discover how you can go from aspiring writer to bestselling author in just six months, with only two hours of weekly effort.

Let us help you unleash your book's potential and leave a lasting legacy.

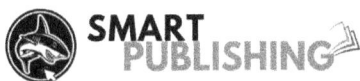

smartpublishingservices.com

www.ingramcontent.com/pod-product-compliance
Lightning Source LLC
Chambersburg PA
CBHW022110280326
41933CB00007B/323